SECOND EDITION

Ross & Wilson

Anatomy
and Physiology
colouring and workbook

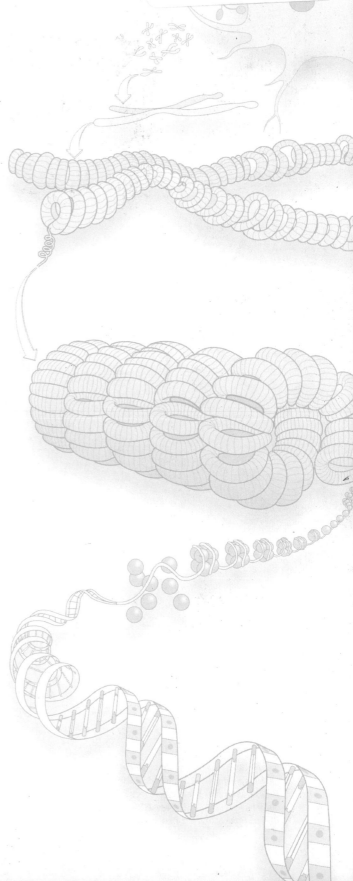

For Churchill Livingstone:

Senior Commissioning Editor: Ninette Premdas
Development Editor: Mairi McCubbin
Project Manager: Frances Affleck
Senior Designer: Sarah Russell
Illustrations Manager: Bruce Hogarth

SECOND EDITION

Ross and Wilson
Anatomy and Physiology
colouring and workbook

Anne Waugh BSc(Hons) MSc CertEd SRN RNT ILTM
Acting Head, School of Acute and Continuing Care Nursing, Napier University, Edinburgh, UK

Allison Grant BSc PhD RGN
Lecturer, School of Biological and Biomedical Sciences, Glasgow Caledonian University, Glasgow, UK

Illustrations by Graeme Chambers

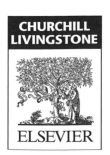

CHURCHILL
LIVINGSTONE

ELSEVIER

EDINBURGH LONDON NEW YORK OXFORD PHILADELPHIA ST LOUIS SYDNEY TORONTO 2006

CHURCHILL LIVINGSTONE
ELSEVIER

© 2004, Elsevier Limited. All rights reserved.
© 2006, Elsevier Science Limited. All rights reserved.

First edition 2004
Second edition 2006

ISBN 10: 0 443 10368 2
ISBN 13: 978 0 443 10368 1

British Library Cataloguing in Publication Data
A catalogue record for this book is available from the British Library

Library of Congress Cataloging in Publication Data
A catalog record for this book is available from the Library of Congress

Notice
Medical knowledge is constantly changing. Standard safety precautions must be followed, but as new research and clinical experience broaden our knowledge, changes in treatment and drug therapy may become necessary or appropriate. Neither the Publisher nor the authors assumes any liability for any injury and/or damage to persons or property arising from this publication.

The Publisher

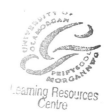
The publisher's policy is to use **paper manufactured from sustainable forests**

Typeset by IMH(Cartrif), Loanhead, Scotland
Printed in Spain

Contents

Preface

Ross and Wilson: Anatomy and Physiology in Health and Illness has been a core text for students for over 40 years. This companion text has been revised to match the new edition of the main text, providing varied learning activities to facilitate and reinforce learning.

The systems approach of the main text forms the framework for the exercises, many of which are based on clear illustrations of body structure and functions. A variety of exercises have been devised to maintain interest and provide choice. The section on 'How to use this book', p. *viii*, explains how the icons and exercises are used in the text.

We hope that you will find this book a stimulating and useful companion to your anatomy and physiology studies, including those times when revision is required. We are always delighted to receive feedback, especially from students, so please continue to send your comments to us via the publishers.

We would have been unable to prepare this book without the help and support of many others, including Graeme Chambers who has patiently revised and created new artwork for this edition. Several people at Churchill Livingstone have also provided encouragement and support and, in particular, we would like to thank Mairi McCubbin and Ninette Premdas for their help during this project.

We would also like to thank our families, Andy, Michael, Seona and Struan for their continuing help and support with this venture.

Edinburgh, 2006   Anne Waugh
                                                                                    Allison Grant

How to use this book
Icons and exercises

 Colouring: identify and colour structures on diagrams.

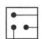 Labelling: identify and label structures on diagrams.

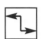 Matching: match statements with reasons; structures with functions; key choices with blanks in a paragraph; and organs on diagrams.

Combinations of these activities are also used to provide variety in the text.

 Multiple-choice questions: identify the correct option from a list of four. Where there is more than one correct option, this is indicated in the question.

 Completion: identify the missing word to complete paragraphs explaining body structure and functions.

 Definitions: explain the meaning of a common anatomical or physiological term.

 Pot luck: a variety of other exercises is also used to facilitate learning. Simple guidance about completion is provided.

1 The body as a whole

The human body is complex, like a highly technical and sophisticated machine. Although it operates as a single entity, it is made up of several parts that work interdependently. This chapter will help you learn about the major systems and control mechanisms that maintain integrated body functioning.

Definitions

Define the following terms:

1. Anatomy _____

   _____.

2. Physiology _____

   _____.

3. Pathology _____

   _____.

LEVELS OF STRUCTURAL COMPLEXITY

 Matching

4. Match the key choices below with the labels on Figure 1.1.

   Key choices:
   System level
   Cellular level
   Organ level
   The human being
   Chemical level
   Tissue level

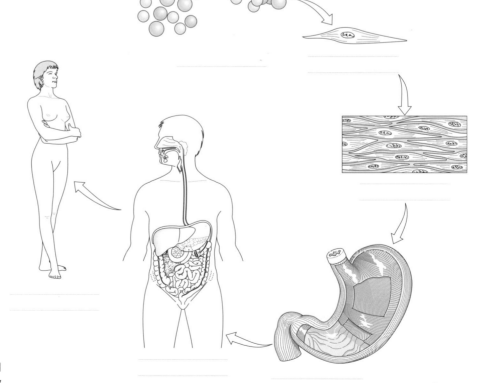

Figure 1.1 The levels of structural complexity

Matching

5. Using the list of key choices on the previous page, complete Table 1.1.

Level of structural complexity	Characteristics
	Comprises many systems that work interdependently to maintain health
	Carry out a specific function and are composed of different types of tissue
	The smallest independent units of living matter
	Consist of one or more organs and contribute to one or more survival needs of the body
	Atoms and molecules that form the building blocks of larger substances
	A group of cells with similar structures and functions

Table 1.1 Levels of structural complexity and their characteristics

THE INTERNAL ENVIRONMENT AND HOMEOSTASIS

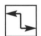 **Matching**

6. Match the key choices listed with the blanks in the paragraph below to describe the internal environment.

Key choices:
Cell membrane	Large
Dry	Skin
External	Small
Internal	Tissue
Interstitial	Watery

The _____ environment surrounds the body and provides the oxygen and nutrients required by all

body cells. The _____ provides a barrier between the _____ external environment and the

_____ internal environment. The _____ environment is the medium in which the body cells exist.

Cells are bathed in fluid called _____ fluid, also known as _____ fluid. The _____

provides a potential barrier to substances entering or leaving cells. This prevents _____ molecules

moving between the cell and interstitial fluid. _____ particles can usually pass through the membrane

more easily and therefore the chemical composition of the fluid inside the cell is different from that outside.

Completion

7. Identify the three components of the negative feedback mechanism in the central heating system shown in Figure 1.2:

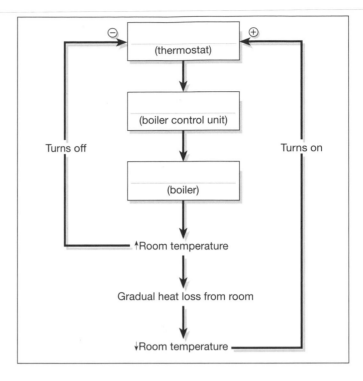

Figure 1.2 Example of a negative feedback mechanism: control of room temperature by a domestic boiler

8. Fill in the blanks in the paragraph below to describe how a negative feedback mechanism operates using body temperature as an example.

The composition of the internal environment is maintained within narrow limits, and this fairly constant state is

called _____. In systems controlled by negative feedback mechanisms, the effector response _____

the effect of the original stimulus. When body temperature falls below the preset level, specialized temperature-

sensitive nerve endings act as _____ and relay this information to cells in the hypothalamus of the brain

that form the _____. This results in activation of _____ responses that raise body

temperature. When body temperature returns to the _____ range again, the temperature-sensitive nerve

endings no longer stimulate the cells in the hypothalamus and the heat conserving mechanisms are switched off.

 ## Pot luck

9. List three responses that will counteract a fall in body temperature:

- _____

- _____

- _____

? Pot luck

10. State three other physiological variables that are controlled by negative feedback:

- _____

- _____

- _____

11. Briefly outline how a positive feedback mechanism operates.

_____

_____

_____

SURVIVAL NEEDS OF THE BODY

? Pot luck

12. Which system is concerned with:

a. Intake of oxygen? _____

b. Intake of nutrients? _____

c. Protection against the external environment? _____.

13. Which system excretes each of the following waste products?

a. Faeces: _____

b. Urine: _____

c. Carbon dioxide: _____.

14. Briefly outline the difference between specific and non-specific defence mechanisms.

_____

_____

_____

_____.

15. True or false? Circle the correct answer for each statement.

a. Most body movement is not under conscious control   **(T/F)**

b. Skeletal muscles move the joints   **(T/ F)**

c. Skeletal muscles are attached to bones by tendons   **(T/F)**.

✎ Completion

16. Complete the paragraph below describing the function of the female reproductive system.

The childbearing years begin at _____ and end at the _____. During this time an _____

matures in the ovary about every _____ days. If _____ takes place it embeds itself in the _____

and grows to maturity during pregnancy, or _____, in about _____ weeks. If fertilization does not occur

it passes out of the body accompanied by bleeding, called _____.

📖 Definitions

Define the following terms:

17. Afferent _____.

18. Efferent _____.

19. Antigen _____.

20. Allergic reaction _____.

▨ ⬑ ⠿ Colouring, matching and labelling

21. Colour and match the following structures on Figure 1.3:

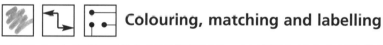

○ Heart
○ Blood vessels

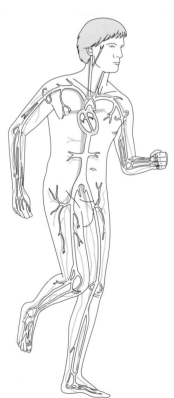

Figure 1.3 The circulatory system

Colouring and labelling

22. Colour and label the following parts of the lymphatic system on Figure 1.4:

| Lymph nodes |
| Lymph vessels |

23. Label the heart on Figure 1.4.

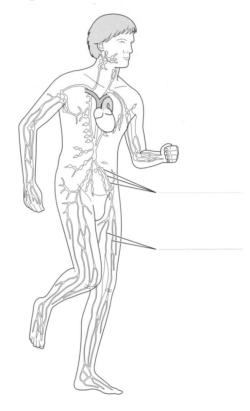

Figure 1.4 The lymphatic system: lymph nodes and vessels

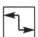 **Colouring, matching and labelling**

24. Colour and match the following parts of the nervous system shown on Figure 1.5:

| ○ Central nervous system |
| ○ Peripheral nervous system |

25. Label the structures indicated on Figure 1.5.

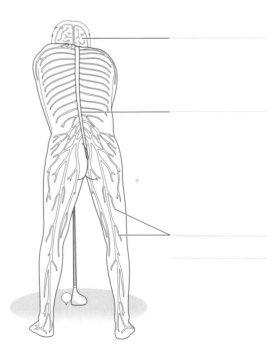

Figure 1.5 The nervous system

Completion

26. Fill in the blanks in the paragraph below to provide an overview of the endocrine system.

The endocrine system consists of a number of _____ in various parts of the body. The glands synthesize and

secrete chemical messengers called _____ into the _____. These chemicals stimulate_____.

Changes in hormone levels are usually controlled by _____ mechanisms. The endocrine system,

in conjunction with part of the _____ system, controls _____ body function. Changes involving the

latter system are usually _____ while those of the endocrine system tend to be _____ and precise.

Completion

27. Complete Table 1.2 by inserting appropriate sensory organ for each of the special senses.

Special sense	Related sensory organ
Sight	
Hearing	
Balance	
Smell	
Taste	

Table 1.2 The special senses and their related sensory organs

Matching and labelling

28. Match the structures listed below with the labels on Figure 1.6:

Bronchus
Lung
Trachea
Larynx
Nasal cavity
Pharynx
Oral cavity

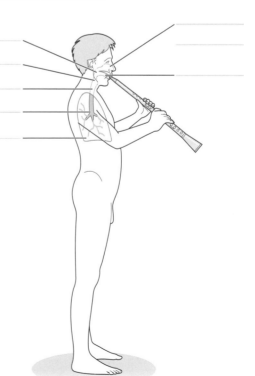

Figure 1.6 The respiratory system

Colouring and labelling

29. Colour and label the organs of the digestive system shown on Figure 1.7.

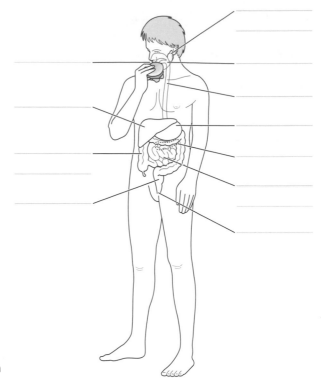

Figure 1.7 The digestive system

30. Colour and label the organs of the urinary system on Figure 1.8:

| Bladder |
| Kidney |
| Urethra |
| Ureter |

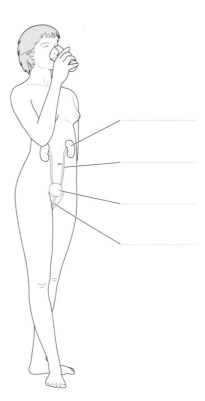

Figure 1.8 The urinary system

Colouring

31. Colour the skeletal muscles on Figure 1.9.

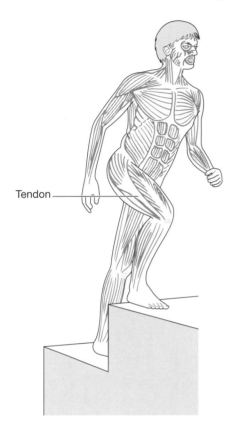

Tendon

Figure 1.9 The skeletal muscles

 Colouring and matching

32. Colour and match the structures listed below with those identified on Figure 1.10:

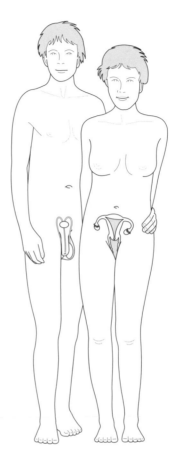

- ○ Vagina
- ○ Ovary
- ○ Uterine tube
- ○ Uterus
- ○ Testis
- ○ Prostate gland
- ○ Penis
- ○ Deferent duct

Figure 1.10 The reproductive systems: male and female

Definitions

Define the following terms:

33. Anabolism _____

_____.

34. Catabolism _____

_____.

35. Micturition _____

_____.

36. Defaecation _____

_____.

Matching

37. Match the items in list A with the definitions in list B.

List A

Acute	Sign
Acquired	Symptom
Chronic	Syndrome
Congenital	

List B

a. An abnormality described by the patient: _____

b. A disorder with which one is born: _____

c. A disorder which develops after birth: _____

d. A long-standing disorder which cannot be cured: _____

e. A collection of signs and symptoms which usually occur together: _____

f. A disease with sudden onset: _____

g. An abnormality seen or measured by people other than the patient: _____.

Definitions

Define the following terms:

38. Aetiology _____
_____.

39. Pathogenesis _____
_____.

40. Prognosis _____
_____.

41. Idiopathic _____
_____.

2 Electrolytes and body fluids

To understand how the tissues, organs and systems of the body work, their fundamental building blocks must be studied. This chapter covers basic chemistry and the structures and functions of important biological molecules.

ATOMS, MOLECULES AND COMPOUNDS

Definitions

Define the following terms:

1. Atom _____

_____.

2. Compound _____

_____.

3. Element _____

_____.

 ### Labelling and completion

4. Figure 2.1 shows the basic structure of an atom. Label the structures shown.

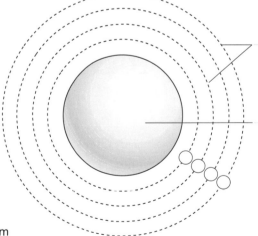

Figure 2.1 The atom

5. Fill in the blank circles to show the maximum number of electrons in each energy level.

Completion

6. Table 2.1 refers to characteristics of the main types of subatomic particle. Complete the table by filling in the blank spaces.

Particle	Mass	Electric charge	Location in atom
Proton			
Neutron			
Electron			

Table 2.1 Characteristics of subatomic particles

 Pot luck

7. Three atoms have electron configurations of 2.8.1., 2.7., and 2.8.18., but only one can be described as stable.

Which one, and why? _____

_____

Definitions

Define the following terms:

8. Atomic number _____

_____.

9. Atomic weight _____

_____.

Completion

10. Complete the grid in Figure 2.2 by filling in the atomic numbers and atomic weights of the atoms shown.

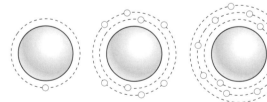

	Hydrogen	Oxygen	Sodium
Atomic number			
Atomic weight			

Figure 2.2 The atomic structures of hydrogen, oxygen and sodium

? MCQs

11. Isotopes are atoms of the same element with different numbers of: _____ .

   a. Protons and electrons   **b.** Electrons   **c.** Neutrons   **d.** Protons and neutrons.

12. Two isotopes of the same element will differ in atomic: _____ .

   a. Charge   **b.** Weight   **c.** Number   **d.** Energy.

✎ Completion

13. Two important types of chemical bond are ionic bonds and covalent bonds. Complete Table 2.2 by ticking the appropriate box for each of the descriptive phrases given.

	Ionic bonds	Covalent bonds
Gives rise to charged particles (ions)		
Commonest bond		
Atoms transfer their electrons		
Links sodium and chloride in a molecule of sodium chloride		
Stable bond		
Atoms share their electrons		
There is no change in the number of protons or neutrons		
The weaker of the two bonds		
Links hydrogen and oxygen in a water molecule		

Table 2.2 Chemical bonds

 Pot luck

14. List three functions of electrolytes:

   • _____

   • _____

   • _____ .

? MCQs

15. An acid solution is characterized by high levels of which ion? _____.

    a. Bicarbonate   **b.** Hydroxyl   **c.** Hydrogen   **d.** Sodium.

16. An alkaline solution is characterized by high levels of which ion? _____.

    a. Bicarbonate   **b.** Hydroxyl   **c.** Hydrogen   **d.** Sodium.

17. Which of the following is true? _____.

    a. An acid solution has a higher pH than an alkaline solution
    b. A strongly acidic solution has a higher pH than a weaker one
    c. There are no ions in a neutral solution
    d. An alkaline solution has a higher pH than an acid one.

18. What is the function of an alkaline buffer in the body? _____

    a. It mops up hydroxyl ions and increases pH   **c.** It mops up hydroxyl ions and decreases pH
    b. It mops up hydrogen ions and decreases pH   **d.** It mops up hydrogen ions and increases pH.

? Pot luck

19. Which two organs are most important in maintaining the acid–base balance in the body by adjusting excretion of excess acid or base?

    • _____

    • _____.

20. Define the term acidosis:

_____

_____.

21. Write down the equation that represents the conversion of carbon dioxide to bicarbonate in body fluids.

_____.

IMPORTANT BIOLOGICAL MOLECULES

 Completion

22. For each of the statements in the left hand column of Table 2.3, decide to which of the classes of biological molecules it belongs (there may be more than one) and tick the appropriate boxes in the table.

	Carbohydrates	Proteins	Nucleotides	Lipids
Building blocks are amino acids				
Contain carbon				
Molecules joined with glycosidic linkages				
Used to build genetic material				
Building blocks are monosaccharides				
Contain glycerol				
Contain hydrogen				
Molecules joined together with peptide bonds				
Strongly hydrophobic				
Built from sugar unit, phosphate group and base				
Enzymes are made from these				
Contain oxygen				

Table 2.3 Characteristics of some important biological molecules

23. Complete the chemical structure in Figure 2.3, which represents a molecule of glucose, by identifying the atoms at the points shown.

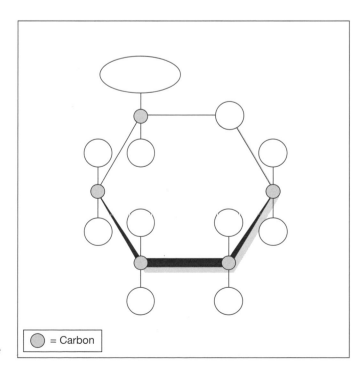

○ = Carbon

Figure 2.3 Structure of a glucose molecule

Pot luck

24. List the four main functions of the carbohydrates.

- _____
- _____
- _____
- _____

 Labelling

25. Figure 2.4 shows the general structure of amino acids, the building block of proteins. Complete it by inserting the appropriate chemical symbols in the spaces provided.

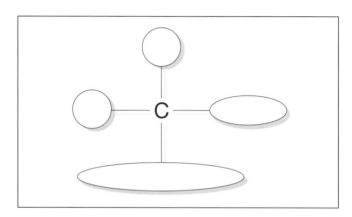

Figure 2.4 Amino acid structure

 Pot luck

26. Proteins are used in the body in many ways. Identify which of the following are composed (at least primarily) of protein by circling the item(s).

Insulin

Haemoglobin

The cell membrane

Glycogen

Vitamin K

Adenosine triphosphate

Deoxyribonucleic acid

Adipose tissue

Antibodies

Enzymes

Sucrose

Collagen

Completion

27. Complete Figure 2.5, which shows the general structure of a fat, by labelling the molecular groups shown.

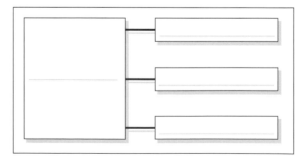

Figure 2.5 General structure of fat

❓ Pot luck

28. The following statements concern the nature and function of lipids. Two are true and two are false. Identify the false statements and write a correct version below.

a. The lipids are a type of fat, and include certain vitamins (e.g. vitamin A) and hormones (e.g. steroids).

_____

_____.

b. The fats provide a source of energy, and excess is stored in the adipose depots of the body.

_____

_____.

c. Phospholipids are an important part of the cell membrane, and form a double layer that helps to regulate the intracellular environment.

_____

_____.

d. Lipid molecules are strongly hydrophilic, meaning water hating, leading to an inability to dissolve in water.

_____

_____.

29. Figure 2.6 shows the structure of ATP and its interconversion with ADP. Label the structures indicated.

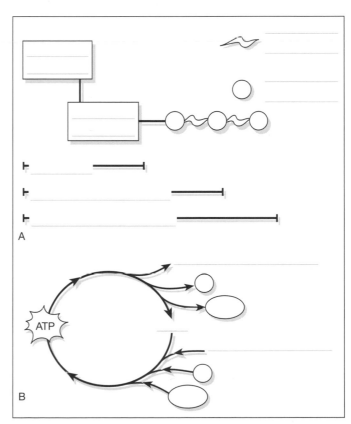

Figure 2.6 ATP and ADP. A. Structures. B. Conversion cycle

Pot luck

30. The following paragraph relates to enzymes, but contains eight errors. Find the errors and correct them.

Enzymes are sugars that are used in the body to slow down the rates of chemical reactions on which the body's metabolism depends. They are themselves normally used up in the reactions they participate in, and are usually fairly specific in the reactions they control. They can either cause two or more molecules to bind together (a catabolic reaction) or cause the breaking up of a molecule into smaller groups (a synthetic reaction). The molecule(s) entering the reaction are called products and they bind to a reactive site on the enzyme molecule called the reaction site. They are bound for only a fraction of a second, but when they are released the reaction has occurred and the new forms of the reactants are now called substrates.

MOVEMENT OF SUBSTANCES WITHIN THE BODY

 MCQs

31. Which of the following is true regarding a substance moving down its concentration gradient? _____.

    a. It requires energy
    b. Diffusion always involves such movement
    c. Substances cannot move down a concentration gradient
    d. It cannot occur across a barrier such as a cell membrane.

32. Which of the following physiological processes involves diffusion? _____.

    a. Gas exchange in the alveoli
    b. Exchange of sodium and potassium ions across cell membranes
    c. Water movement in and out of cells
    d. Movement of molecules that requires a supply of ATP.

33. Movement of water molecules occurs by:_____.

    a. Diffusion   **b.** Active transport   **c.** Dilution   **d.** Osmosis.

34. Which of the following statements regarding water movement is true (choose all that apply)? _____.

    a. A hypertonic solution contains more solute (dissolved particles) than a hypotonic one
    b. Water moves from a hypotonic solution into a hypertonic solution (assuming no barrier to water movement exists)
    c. Red blood cells placed in a beaker of pure water will shrink because water will leave the cells across the semipermeable cell membrane
    d. If two solutions on either side of a semipermeable membrane are isotonic to each other, it means no net movement of water molecules will occur.

BODY FLUIDS

 Pot luck

35. What percentage of body mass in an average adult is water? _____

36. Which of the following is associated primarily with the intracellular environment (circle all that apply)?

Sodium	Urine
Cytoplasm	Glomerular filtrate
Cerebrospinal fluid	Lymph
Synovial fluid	Potassium
Plasma	Blood
Saliva	ATP

3 The cells, tissues, organization of the body

Cells are the smallest functional units of the body. Groups of similar cells form tissues, each of which has a distinct and specialized function. This chapter will help you learn about the structure of cells and characteristics of different types of tissue. The last section considers the organization of the body including anatomical terminology, the skeleton and the body cavities.

THE CELL: STRUCTURE AND FUNCTIONS

  Colouring and labelling

1. Colour and label the intracellular organelles identified on Figure 3.1.

2. Label the plasma membrane on Figure 3.1.

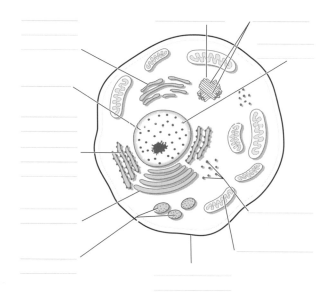

Figure 3.1 The simple cell

 Matching

3. Match the organelles from the list of key choices below with their functions in Table 3.1:

Key choices:	
Lysosomes	Microfilaments
Ribsomes	Microtubules
Nucleus	Golgi apparatus
Smooth endoplasmic reticulum	Mitochondria
Rough endoplasmic reticulum	

Organelle	Function
nucleus	The largest organelle, directs the activities of the cell
mit	Sausage-shaped structures, often described as the powerhouse of the cell. Sites of aerobic respiration
riba	Tiny granules consisting of RNA and protein that synthesize proteins for use within cells
	Proteins exported from cells are manufactured here
	Lipids and steroid hormones are synthesized here
	Stacks of closely flattened membranous sacs that form membrane-bound granules called secretory vesicles
	Secretory granules that contain enzymes for the breakdown of large cellular wastes, e.g. fragments of old organelles
	The tiny strands of protein that provide the structural support and shape of a cell
	Contractile proteins involved in movement of cells and of organelles within cells

Table 3.1 Intracellular organelles and their functions

Pot luck

4. There are four errors in the paragraph below describing the structure of cell membranes. Find the errors and correct them.

The plasma membrane consists of two layers of phospholipids with some carbohydrate molecules embedded in them. The phospholipid molecules have a head which is electrically charged and hydrophilic (meaning water hating) and a tail that has no charge and is hydrophobic. The phospholipid bilayer is arranged like a sandwich with the hydrophilic heads on the inside and the hydrophobic tails on the outside. These differences influence the passage of substances across the membrane.

 Completion

5. The paragraph below describes the structure and function of the nucleus. Complete the paragraph by filling in the blanks.

Most body cells have one nucleus. Exceptions are mature _____ cells, which have none, and _____ cells that may have several. The nucleus is contained within the _____, a membrane that has _____, which allow passage of substances between the nucleus and the_____. It contains the body's _____ material, which consists of 46 _____ that are built from _____.

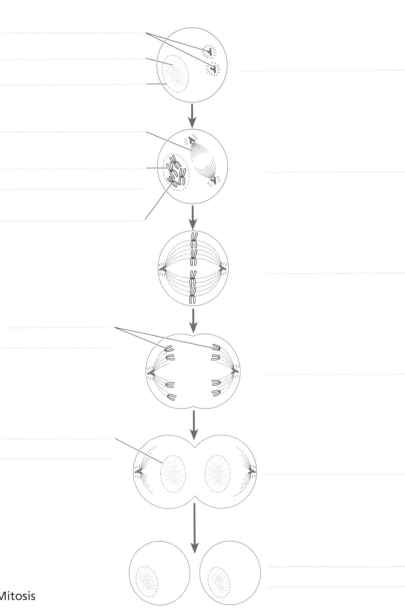

  Labelling and colouring

6. Label the stages of mitosis on Figure 3.2.

7. Colour the genetic material shown on the parts of Figure 3.2.

8. Label the cellular structures seen on light microscopy during mitosis.

Figure 3.2 Mitosis

? Pot luck

9. Identify whether the statements below are true or false.

    a. Chromatids are visible on microscopy during interphase. **(T/F)**

    b. Centrioles are visible on microscopy during interphase. **(T/F)**

    c. Each chromosome consists of two centromeres. **(T/F)**

    d. Mitosis results in four daughter cells. **(T/F)**

    e. The daughter cells of mitosis have 23 chromosomes. **(T/F)**

    f. The daughter cells of mitosis are genetically identical. **(T/F)**

Definitions

Define the following terms:

10. Active transport _____

_____.

11. Passive transport _____

_____.

? MCQs

12. The energy for active transport comes from: _____.

    a. RNA   **b.** ATP   **c.** DNA   **d.** ADP.

13. Movement of substances against their concentration gradient is known as: _____.

    a. Active transport   **b.** Osmosis   **c.** Diffusion   **d.** Filtration.

14. Osmosis is movement of: _____.

    a. Any substance down its concentration gradient   **c.** Water up its concentration gradient
    b. Any substance up its concentration gradient   **d.** Water down its concentration gradient.

15. The sodium pump is an example of: _____.

    a. Active transport   **b.** Osmosis   **c.** Diffusion   **d.** Filtration.

16. The transport maximum occurs when there are a finite number of carriers to transport a substance across cell membranes and determines the maximum rate of: _____.

    a. Filtration   **b.** Facilitated diffusion   **c.** Osmosis   **d.** Diffusion.

17. Diffusion is movement of: _____.

    a. Water up its concentration gradient   **c.** Any substance down its concentration gradient
    b. Water down its concentration gradient   **d.** Any substance up its concentration gradient.

Matching

18. Match the key choices to the spaces in the paragraph below to describe bulk transport.

Key choices:
Key choices:
Exocytosis
Digest
Pinocytosis
Vacuole
Phagocytosis
Plasma membrane
Enzymes
Lysosomes.

Transfer of large particles across the plasma membrane into the cell occurs by _____ and _____. The particles are engulfed by extensions of the _____ that enclose them forming a membrane-bound _____.

Then _____ adhere to the cell membrane releasing _____ that _____ the contents. Extrusion of waste materials by the reverse process is called _____.

TISSUES

   Colouring, matching and labelling

19. Name the types of epithelial tissues shown in Figure 3.3.

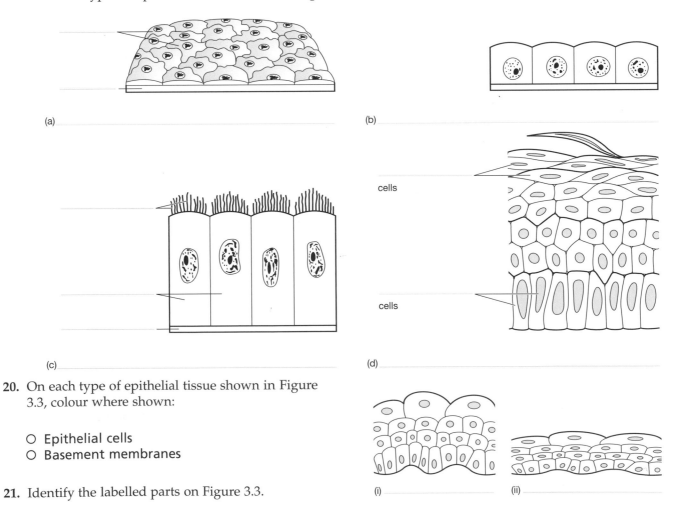

(a) _____

(b) _____

cells

cells

(c) _____

(d) _____

20. On each type of epithelial tissue shown in Figure 3.3, colour where shown:

○ Epithelial cells
○ Basement membranes

21. Identify the labelled parts on Figure 3.3.

(i) _____

(ii) _____

(e) _____

Figure 3.3 Types of epithelial tissue

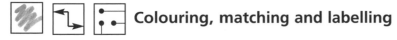 **Colouring, matching and labelling**

22. Name each type of connective tissue shown in Figure 3.4.

23. Colour the matrix on each part of Figure 3.4.

24. Label the cells and fibres on each part of Figure 3.4.

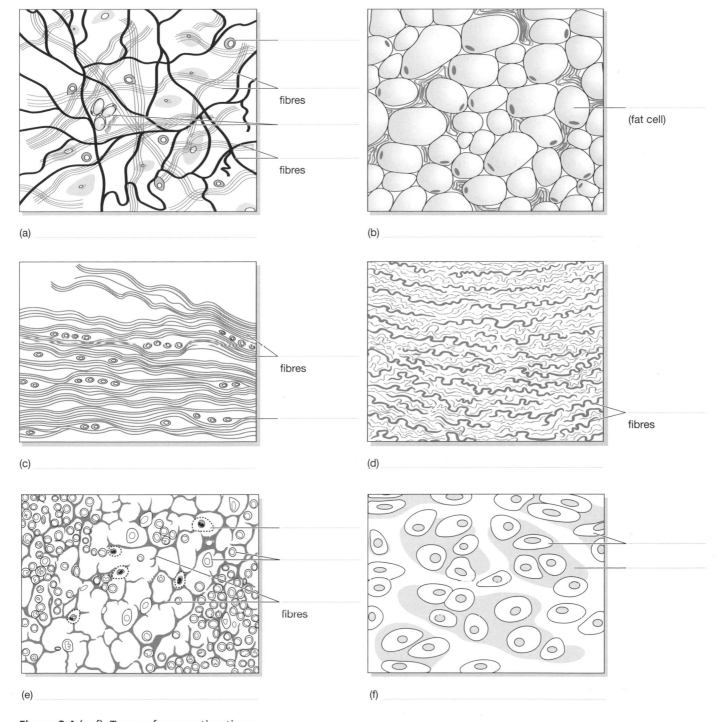

(a) _____ (b) _____

(c) _____ (d) _____

(e) _____ (f) _____

fibres

(fat cell)

fibres

fibres

fibres

Figure 3.4 (a–f) Types of connective tissue

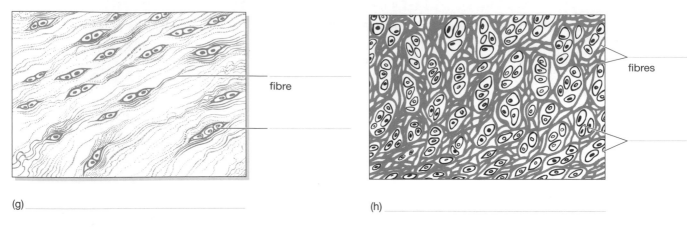

(g) _____   (h) _____

Figure 3.4 (g–h) Types of connective tissue

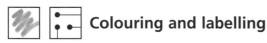 **Colouring and labelling**

25. Name the types of muscle tissue shown in Figure 3.5 and note the differences.

26. Colour the nuclei on the muscle tissue shown in Figure 3.5.

27. Label an intercalated disc on Figure 3.5.

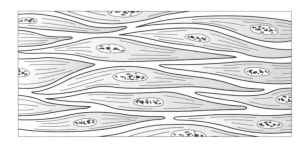

B. _____

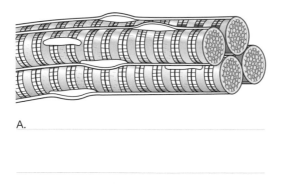

A. _____

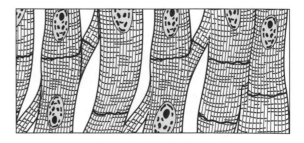

C. _____

Figure 3.5 Types of muscle tissue

Completion

28. Complete the blanks in the paragraph below to describe the structure and functions of muscle tissue.

Muscle cells are also called _____. Muscle tissue has the property of _____ that brings about movement, both within the body and of the body itself. This requires a blood supply to provide _____, _____ and _____, and to remove _____. The chemical energy needed is derived from _____.

    Skeletal muscle is also known as _____ muscle because _____ is under conscious control. When examined under the microscope, the cells are roughly _____ in shape and may be as long as _____ cm. The cells show a pattern of clearly visible stripes, also known as _____. Skeletal muscle is stimulated by _____ impulses that originate in the brain or spinal cord and end at the _____.

    Smooth muscle has the intrinsic ability to _____ and _____, but it can also be stimulated by _____ impulses, some _____ and _____.

    Cardiac muscle is found only in the wall of the _____, which has its own _____ system, meaning that this tissue contracts in a co-ordinated manner without external stimulation. _____ impulses and some _____ influence activity of this type of muscle.

? MCQs

29. Which of the following is not a function of skeletal muscle? _____.

   a. Generation of heat   **b.** Enabling movement   **c.** Peristalsis   **d.** Maintaining posture.

30. The characteristics of cardiac muscle include (choose all that apply): _____.

   a. Branching cells   **b.** Intercalated discs   **c.** Cross stripes   **d.** Spindle-shaped cells.

31. Smooth muscle may also be described as (choose all that apply): _____.

   a. Non-striated   **b.** Active   **c.** Involuntary   **d.** Skeletal.

32. Smooth muscle is found in (choose all that apply): _____.

   a. The heart   **b.** Blood vessel walls   **c.** Ducts of glands   **d.** The urinary bladder.

Completion

33. Complete the paragraphs below to describe characteristics of membranes.

Mucous membrane is sometimes referred to as the _____. It forms the moist lining of body tracts, e.g. the

_____, _____ and _____ tracts. The membrane consists of _____ cells, some of

which produce a secretion called _____. This sticky substance protects the lining from _____. In the

alimentary tract it _____ the contents and in the respiratory system it traps _____.

     A serous membrane may also be known as the _____. It consists of a double layer of _____

connective tissue lined by _____ epithelium. The layer lining the body cavity is the _____ layer

and that surrounding organs within a cavity, the _____ layer. There are three sites where serous

membranes are found:

     a. the _____ lining the thoracic cavity and surrounding the lungs

     b. the _____ lining the pericardial cavity and surrounding the heart

     c. the _____ lining the abdominal cavity and surrounding the abdominal organs.
     Synovial membrane lines the cavities of _____. It consists of _____ tissue

containing _____ fibres. This membrane secretes a clear, sticky, oily substance known as _____. It

provides _____ and _____, and prevents _____ between structures in _____ joints.

Colouring, matching and labelling

34. Distinguish the exocrine glands on Figure 3.6
     by colouring:

     ○ Simple glands
     ○ Compound glands

35. Name the different types of exocrine glands on
     Figure 3.6.

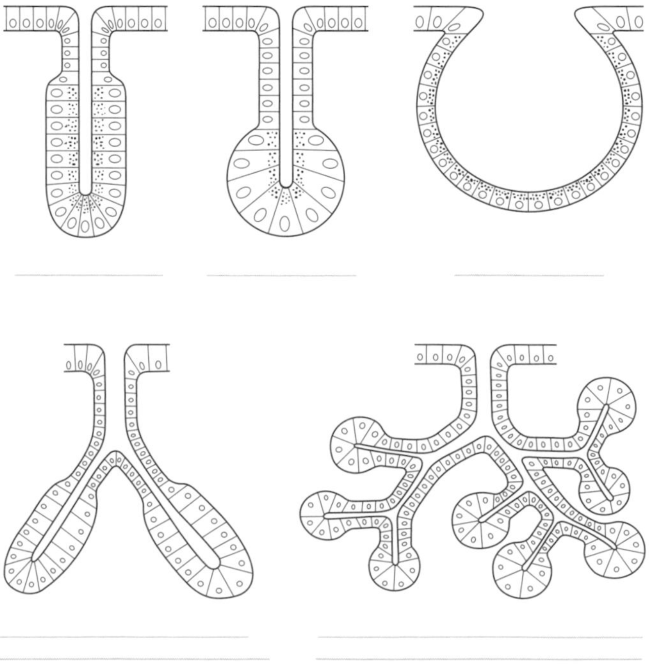

Figure 3.6 Exocrine glands

ORGANIZATION OF THE BODY

 Pot luck

36. The sentence below describes the position assumed in all anatomical descriptions to ensure accuracy and consistency. There are five errors in the sentence. Please correct them to describe the anatomical position.

The body is in the horizontal position with the head facing upwards, the arms facing outwards with the palms of the hands facing downwards and the feet apart.

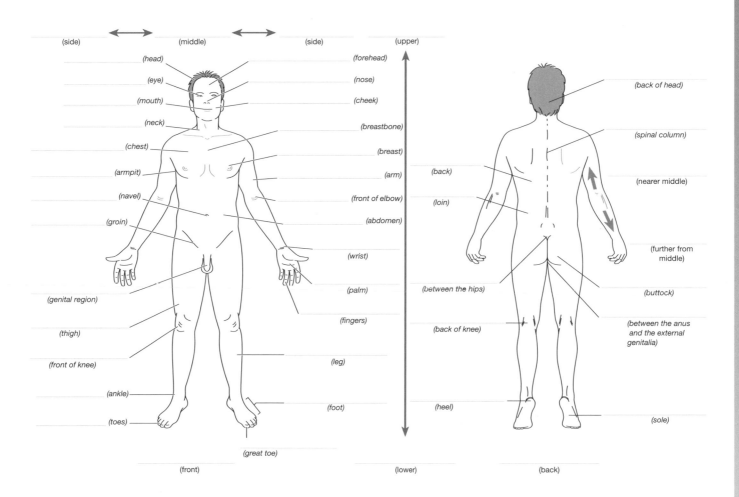

Figure 3.7 Regional and directional terms

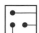 **Labelling**

37. Identify the regional terms indicated on Figure 3.7.

38. Label the directional terms indicated on Figure 3.7.

Colouring, matching and labelling

39. Colour and match the following parts of the skeleton in Figure 3.8:

> ○ Axial skeleton
> ○ Appendicular skeleton

40. Label the bones identified on Figure 3.8.

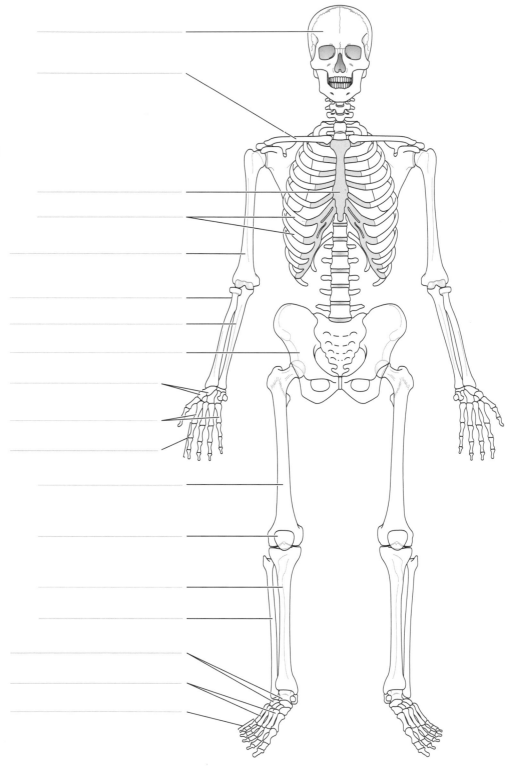

Figure 3.8 The skeleton

Colouring and labelling

41. Colour and label the following bones of the cranium and face on Figure 3.9:

Temporal bone	Vomer
Occipital bone	Nasal bone
Parietal bone	Ethmoid bone
Frontal bone	Maxilla
Sphenoid bone	Palatine bone

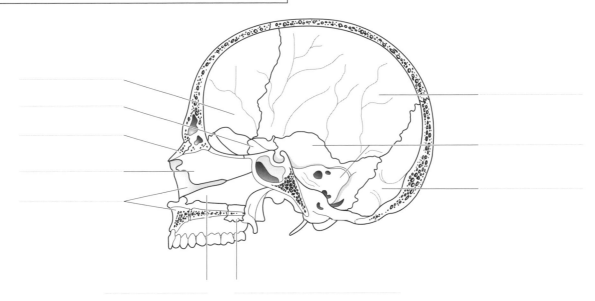

Figure 3.9 The bones forming the cranium and face – viewed from the left

 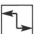 **Colouring and matching**

42. Colour and match the following parts of Figure 3.10:

○ Intercostal muscles
○ Sternocleidomastoid muscles
○ Diaphragm
○ Ribs
○ Vertebrae
○ Sternum
○ Clavicles
○ Costal cartilages

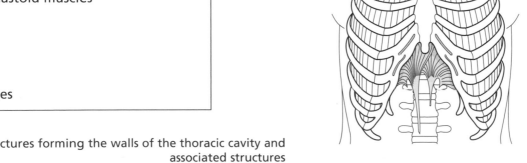

Figure 3.10 Structures forming the walls of the thoracic cavity and associated structures

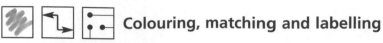 **Colouring, matching and labelling**

43. Colour and match the following structures found within the posterior abdominal cavity on Figure 3.11:

○ Spleen
○ Right adrenal gland
○ Kidneys
○ Ureters
○ Inferior vena cava
○ Aorta

44. Colour and label the other organs identified on Figure 3.11.

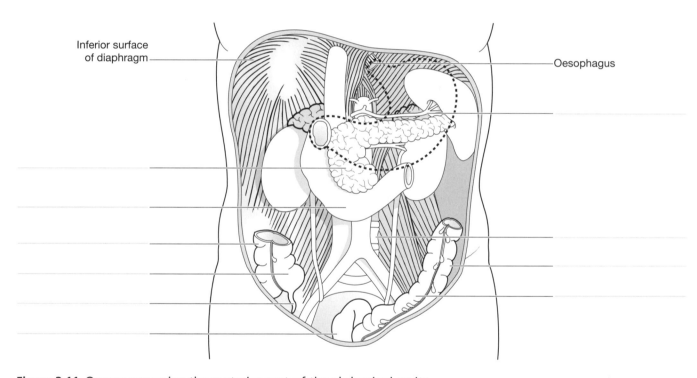

Inferior surface of diaphragm

Oesophagus

Figure 3.11 Organs occupying the posterior part of the abdominal cavity

Labelling

45. Identify the nine regions of the abdominal cavity shown in Figure 3.12.

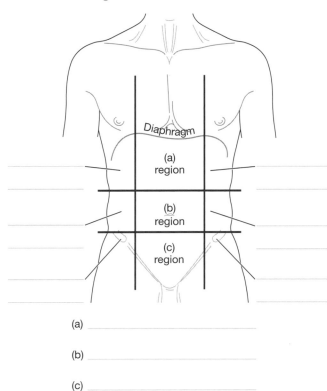

(a) _____

(b) _____

(c) _____

Figure 3.12 Regions of the abdominal cavity

Applying what you know

46. For each organ in list A, state in which body region(s) in List B the organ is situated:

List A

a. Brain: _____.

b. Stomach: _____.

c. Small intestine: _____.

d. Large intestine: _____.

e. Lungs: _____.

f. Liver: _____.

g. Rectum: _____.

h. Bladder: _____.

i. Heart: _____.

List B

1. Hypogastric region
2. Right lumbar region
3. Epigastric region
4. Left iliac region
5. None of these.

47. State which body cavity a surgeon would open to operate on the:

a. Appendix: _____.

b. Heart: _____.

c. Uterus: _____.

d. Stomach: _____.

e. Brain: _____.

f. Rectum: _____.

g. Lungs: _____.

h. Spleen: _____.

Definitions

Define the following terms:

48. Carcinogen _____
_____.

49. Tumour _____
_____.

4 The blood

The blood is a fluid connective tissue, which travels within the closed circulatory system. It carries nutrients, wastes, respiratory gases and other substances important to body function. This chapter will test your understanding of the physiology of blood.

COMPOSITION OF BLOOD

  Labelling and colouring

1. Figure 4.1A shows whole blood that has been prevented from clotting and allowed to stand for some time. Label and colour the two layers shown.

2. Figure 4.1B shows whole blood that has been allowed to clot. Label and colour the parts shown.

3. What is present in the fluid portion in Figure 4.1A that is absent in Figure 4.1B? _____.

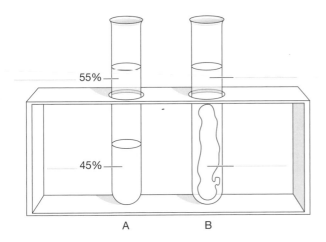

A   B

Figure 4.1 The proportions of blood cells and plasma in whole blood separated by gravity. A. Blood prevented from clotting. B. Blood allowed to clot

These chemicals travel from the gland of origin to distant tissues	
These provide the building blocks for new tissue proteins	
These molecules combat antigens	
90–92% of plasma is this	
This substance is needed for haemoglobin synthesis	
An important respiratory waste is carried as this	
This participates in the clotting reaction	
This is needed for healthy bones and teeth	
This is the principal fuel source for the tissues	
This is a nitrogenous waste	

Table 4.1 Components of plasma

 Matching

4. Table 4.1 lists various descriptive phrases. Match them with the suggested components of plasma in list A below. (Be careful, not everything in list A is actually found in plasma!)

List A
Urea   Hormones
Haemoglobin   Water
Amino acids   Albumin
Fibrinogen   Bile
Glucose   Antibodies
Rhesus antigens   Bicarbonate ion
Intrinsic factor   Iron
Phosphate

MCQs

5. Which of the following is responsible for keeping plasma fluid within blood vessels? _____.

   a. Hydrostatic pressure   **b.** Osmotic pressure   **c.** Blood pressure   **d.** Pulse pressure.

6. Which of the following plasma proteins is mainly responsible for exerting the pressure that keeps plasma fluid within blood vessels? _____.

   a. Thyroglobulin   **b.** Immunoglobulin   **c.** Fibrinogen   **d.** Albumin.

7. Which is the most abundant plasma protein? _____.

   a. Thyroglobulin   **b.** Immunoglobulin   **c.** Fibrinogen   **d.** Albumin.

8. Which of the following plasma proteins is involved in neutralizing antigens? _____.

   a. Thyroglobulin   **b.** Immunoglobulin   **c.** Fibrinogen   **d.** Albumin.

9. Which of the following are transport proteins (choose all that apply)? _____.

   a. Thyroglobulin   **b.** Immunoglobulin   **c.** Fibrinogen   **d.** Albumin.

10. Which of the following is involved in blood clotting? _____.

    a. Thyroglobulin   **b.** Immunoglobulin   **c.** Fibrinogen   **d.** Albumin

CELLULAR CONTENT OF BLOOD

 Colouring and labelling

11. Figure 4.2 shows the eight main types of blood cell. Name each type in the space provided.

12. In Figure 4.2, colour the granules in the cytoplasm of those white cells that contain them and the nuclei of the cells that have them.

13. The term used to describe blood cell formation is:

    _____.

 Pot luck

14. Explain why cell (a) has no nucleus.

    _____.

15. List three substances that are found within the cytoplasmic granules of cells (c), (d) and (e).

    _____.

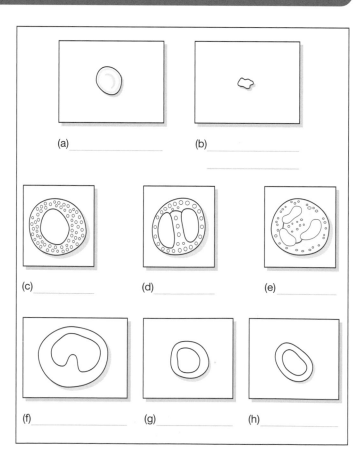

Figure 4.2 Blood cells

Matching

16. The letters in list A correspond with the blood cells in Figure 4.2. The box below lists 20 numbered key choices that can be used to describe each of them. Match each cell type with the relevant key choices. (Be careful, you can use each key choice more than once!)

List A. List the numbers of the key choices here.

a: _____

b: _____

c: _____

d: _____

e: _____

f: _____

g: _____

h: _____

Key choices:
1. Circulating mast cell
2. Makes antibodies
3. Important in clotting
4. Granulocyte
5. Agranulocyte
6. Commonest blood phagocyte
7. 1–6% of total white blood cells
8. Cell fragment
9. Large single nucleus
10. Involved in immunity
11. Diameter of about 7 microns
12. Has no nucleus
13. Contain haemoglobin
14. $0.04–0.44 \times 10^9$ cells/litre
15. Smallest white blood cell(s)
16. 2–10% of total white cells
17. Made in red bone marrow
18. Originate from pluripotent stem cells
19. Synthesis is called erythropoiesis
20. Biconcave in shape

? **MCQs**

17. How long does it take to make a red blood cell? _____.

    a. 7 hours   **b.** 7 days   **c.** 3 hours   **d.** 3 weeks.

18. Which two substances are necessary for normal red blood cell maturation? _____.

    a. Intrinsic factor and folic acid   **c.** Folic acid and iron
    b. Iron and vitamin B_{12} **d.** Folic acid and vitamin B_{12}.

19. Where in the body is oxyhaemoglobin formed? _____.

    a. In the lungs   **b.** In the kidneys   **c.** In the heart   **d.** In the brain.

20. Which of the following best describes the function of haemoglobin? _____.

    a. Supply of oxygen to the tissues   **c.** Iron transport in the blood
    b. To give red blood cells their colour   **d.** Carriage of respiratory gases.

21. If a haemoglobin molecule is *saturated*, which of the following would be true? _____.

    a. All six of its oxygen binding sites are full
    b. The haemoglobin molecule is carrying its full complement of iron
    c. It has collected carbon dioxide in the tissues and has changed from bright red to bluish in colour
    d. The molecule is likely to be in the pulmonary vein rather than in a systemic vein.

22. Which of the following would decrease the release of oxygen from oxyhaemoglobin? _____.

    a. Increased tissue metabolism
    b. Reduced tissue temperature
    c. Increased tissue carbon dioxide production
    d. Reduced red blood cell numbers.

Matching

23. Figure 4.3 is a flow chart describing red blood cell synthesis. Complete it by putting the statements below into the diagram in the right order.

Bone marrow increases erythropoiesis

Increased blood oxygen-carrying capacity reverses tissue hypoxia

Red blood cell numbers rise

Kidneys secrete erythropoietin into the blood

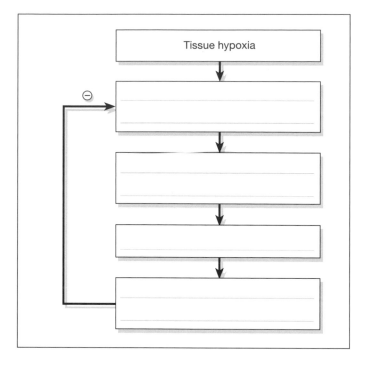

Figure 4.3 Control of erythropoiesis

Completion

24. The following paragraph describes the destruction of red blood cells. Complete it by filling in the blanks.

The life span of red blood cells is usually about _____ days. Their breakdown, also called _____, is carried out by phagocytic _____ cells found mainly in the _____, _____ and _____. Their breakdown releases the mineral _____, which is kept by the body and stored in the _____. It is used to form new _____. The protein released is converted to the intermediate _____, and then to the yellow pigment _____, before being bound to plasma protein and transported to the _____, where it is excreted in the _____.

25. Complete Table 4.2, which describes the ABO system of blood grouping.

Blood group	Type of antigen present on red cell surface	Type of antibody present in plasma	Can safely donate to:	Can safely receive from:
A				
B				
AB				
O				

Table 4.2 The ABO system of blood grouping

26. Which of the blood groups in Table 4.2 is known as the universal donor? _____.

27. Which of these blood groups is known as the universal recipient? _____.

28. Complete Table 4.3, which describes the function of the main white blood cells, by ticking the appropriate boxes against each cell type.

	Neutrophils	Eosinophils	Basophils	Monocytes	Lymphocytes
Phagocyte					
Involved in allergy					
Converted to macrophages					
Release histamine					
Many in lymph nodes					
Kupffer cells					
Increased numbers in infections					
Kill parasites					
Part of the reticuloendothelial system					

Table 4.3 Characteristics of white blood cells

29. Blood clotting is a complex process, but it can be divided conveniently into four main stages. For each of the headings below, outline the main events as the clot is formed and then broken down.

a. Vasoconstriction

_____

_____

_____

b. Platelet plug formation

_____

_____

_____

c. Coagulation

_____

_____

_____

d. Fibrinolysis

_____

_____

_____.

5 The cardiovascular system

The cardiovascular system consists of the heart, which is a pump, and the vast network of vessels, which are the transport system for the blood. Together, they supply all the body's tissues with nutrients and carry away wastes. This chapter will help you to understand its structure, the functions of the heart and the different types of blood vessel, and the control of blood pressure. The lymphatic system, which is also important in fluid transport, is dealt with in a separate chapter.

BLOOD VESSELS

 Completion

1. Complete the following paragraph, which describes the two circulation systems of the blood, by inserting the correct word in the spaces provided.

The heart pumps blood into two separate circulatory systems, the _____ circulation and the

_____ circulation. The _____ side of the heart pumps blood to the lungs, whereas the _____

side of the heart supplies the rest of the body. The _____ are the sites of exchange of nutrients, gases and

wastes. Tissue wastes, including carbon dioxide, pass into the _____ and the tissues are supplied with

_____ and _____.

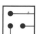 **Completion and labelling**

2. Figure 5.1 illustrates the principal components of the cardiovascular system. Name the structures to which the following letters correspond.

a. _____

b. _____

c. _____

d. _____.

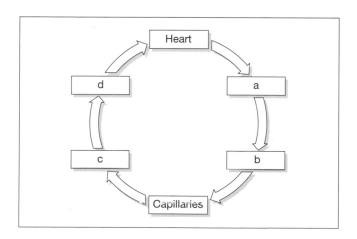

Figure 5.1 The relationship between the heart and different types of blood vessel

Labelling and colouring

3. Label and colour Figure 5.2.

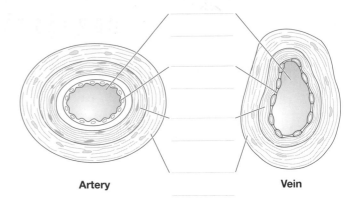

Figure 5.2 Structures of an artery and a vein

Artery   Vein

 Completion

4. Match each of the three layers you identified in Figure 5.2 with the two most appropriate descriptive phrases given in Table 5.1.

Descriptive phrase	Layer (tunica) of vessel wall
Squamous epithelium	
Contains mainly fibrous tissue	
Endothelial layer	
Consists partly of muscle tissue	
The vessel's elastic tissue is here	
Outer layer	

Table 5.1 Layers of vessel wall

? MCQs

5. Veins have thinner walls than arteries because they: _____.

    a. Carry less blood than arteries
    b. Carry blood at lower pressures than arteries
    c. Unlike arteries, have no muscle in their walls
    d. Are the vessels where gas and nutrient exchange takes place.

6. Collateral circulation is: _____.

    a. Lymphatic vessels running alongside arteries
    b. Venous drainage from the tissues
    c. The relationship of the systemic and pulmonary circuits
    d. More than one artery supplying an area.

7. What is the function of valves in blood vessels? _____.

    a. To keep the blood flowing in one direction
    b. To control the rate of blood flowing back to the heart
    c. To support the blood vessel walls
    d. To shut off blood flow in a damaged vessel.

8. Valves are formed from which kind(s) of tissue (choose all that apply)? _____.

    a. Muscle   **b.** Adipose   **c.** Endothelial   **d.** Connective.

Completion

9. Complete the following paragraph by inserting the correct term in the blanks provided.

The smallest arterioles split up into a large number of tinier vessels called _____. Across the walls of these vessels, the tissues obtain _____ and _____, and get rid of their _____. The walls of these vessels are therefore thin, being only _____ thick. Substances such as _____ and _____ can pass across them, whereas larger constituents of blood such as _____ and _____ are retained within the vessel. This vast network of microscopic vessels have a diameter of only about _____, and link the arterioles to the _____. In some parts of the body, such as the liver, the vessels in the tissues are wider than this, and are called _____. Blood flow here is _____ than in other tissues because of the bigger lumen.

? **Pot luck**

10. Decide whether the following terms apply to vasoconstriction or vasodilation.

 a. Vessel wall thins: _____.

 b. Volume of blood that is carried is increased: _____.

 c. Usually caused by sympathetic stimulation: _____.

 d. Decreased resistance to blood flow: _____.

 e. Smooth muscle in vessel wall is contracted: _____.

 f. Usually follows a decrease in sympathetic stimulation: _____.

 g. Lumen of vessel is wider: _____.

 h. Vessel wall thickens: _____.

 i. Smooth muscle in vessel wall is relaxed: _____.

 j. Lumen of vessel is reduced: _____.

 k. Increased resistance to blood flow: _____.

 l. Volume of blood that is carried is decreased: _____.

? **MCQs**

11. Internal respiration is the: _____.

 a. Supply of oxygen and nutrients to blood vessel walls by the vasa vasorum
 b. Breakdown of oxyhaemoglobin in the tissues to release oxygen
 c. Exchange of carbon dioxide and oxygen between blood and tissue cells
 d. Accumulation of wastes in the tissues that increases oxygen release to the cells.

12. Which of the following does not represent an example of autoregulation? _____.

 a. Control of blood vessel diameter by the vasomotor centre in the medulla oblongata
 b. Vasodilation in leg muscles following a 10 mile run
 c. Increased blood supply to an area of inflammation after tissue injury
 d. Rebound increase in blood supply to an organ following a period of hypoxia.

13. Which of the following does not represent a mechanism of carbon dioxide transport in the blood? _____ .

   a. Bound to haemoglobin   **b.** As bicarbonate ions   **c.** Dissolved in blood water   **d.** As hydrogen ions.

14. Flow along a blood vessel is determined in health primarily by: _____ .

   a. Blood vessel length
   b. Blood vessel diameter
   c. Blood viscosity
   d. Blood volume.

Matching

15. Substances moving in and out of capillaries do so usually by one of the following processes: osmosis, diffusion or active transport. Decide whether the following statements apply to any one or any combination of these three, and complete Table 5.2 by ticking in the appropriate columns.

	Osmosis	Diffusion	Active transport
Movement only down a concentration gradient			
Movement of water molecules			
Movement across a semipermeable membrane			
Movement requires energy			
Movement up a concentration gradient possible			
Movement does not require energy			
Movement of oxygen			
Movement of carbon dioxide			

Table 5.2 Characteristics of osmosis, diffusion and active transport

16. For each of the five statements in list A, identify the most appropriate answer from list B. (You may need the items in list B more than once.)

List A

a. Plasma proteins in the bloodstream are responsible for exerting _____ .

b. The hydrostatic pressure of the blood is also known as _____ .

c. The main force opposing the osmotic pressure of the blood is _____ .

d. The main force pushing fluid out of the arterial end of the capillary is the _____ .

e. The main force drawing fluid back into the venous end of the capillary is the _____ .

> *List B*
> Hydrostatic pressure
> Blood pressure
> Osmotic pressure

Matching and colouring

17. Figure 5.3 shows the effect of capillary pressures on water movement in and out of the capillary. Using different colours, colour and match the arrows to represent hydrostatic and osmotic pressures at each end of the capillary.

○ Hydrostatic pressure
○ Osmotic pressure

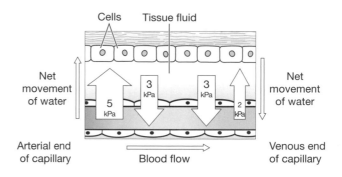

Figure 5.3 Effect of capillary pressures on water movement between capillaries and cells

THE HEART

  ## Colouring and labelling

18. Label Figure 5.4.

19. On Figure 5.4, colour the vessels carrying oxygenated blood red and the vessels carrying deoxygenated blood blue.

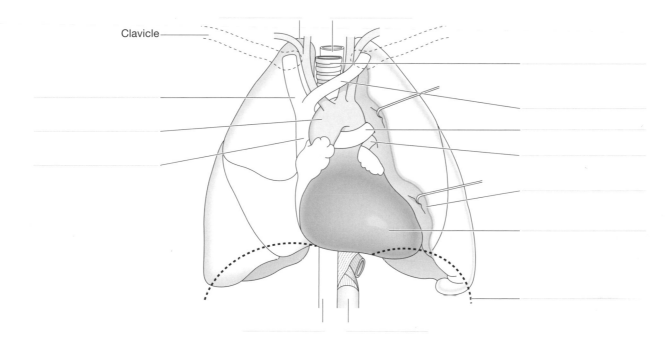

Figure 5.4 Organs associated with the heart

Colouring and labelling

20. Figure 5.5 shows the main layers of the heart wall.
    Colour and label the structures shown.

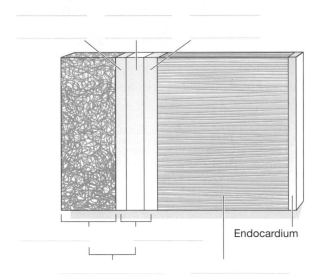

Endocardium

Figure 5.5 Layers of the heart wall

? MCQs

21. Which layer of the heart wall lines its chambers? _____.

    a. Myocardium   **b.** Serous pericardium   **c.** Endocardium   **d.** Parietal pericardium.

22. Which layer of the heart wall contains muscle? _____.

    a. Myocardium   **b.** Visceral pericardium   **c.** Fibrous pericardium   **d.** Endocardium.

23. The pericardial space lies between which layers of the heart wall? _____.

    a. The myocardium and the endocardium
    b. The fibrous pericardium and the serous pericardium
    c. The endocardium and the fibrous pericardium
    d. The visceral pericardium and the parietal pericardium.

24. Pericardial fluid is secreted by the: _____.

    a. Endocardium   **b.** Serous pericardium   **c.** Fibrous pericardium   **d.** Myocardium.

⬉ Matching

25. Match each of the statements in list A with the appropriate item in list B. (You will need to use the items in list B more than once.)

List A

a. Junctions between the cells are called intercalated discs: _____.

b. Secretes pericardial fluid: _____.

c. Fibrous and inelastic tissue: _____.

d. Made up of endothelial cells: _____.

e. Is a double membrane, folded back on itself: _____.

f. Prevents the heart from overdistension: _____.

g. Covers the valves of the heart: _____.

h. The muscle here is found only in the heart: _____.

i. Contains the pericardial space: _____.

j. Thickest in the left ventricle, and at the base of the heart: _____.

k. Continuous with the lining of the blood vessels leaving and entering the heart: _____.

List B
Myocardium
Endocardium
Fibrous pericardium
Serous pericardium

---

26. The double membrane arrangement of the serous pericardium is found in which two other locations in the body?

- _____

- _____.

Labelling

27. Name the chambers of the heart shown on Figure 5.6.

A:	B:
C:	D:

28. Label all the structures indicated on Figure 5.6.

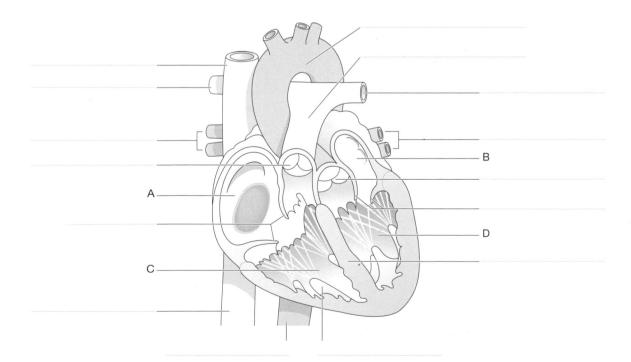

Figure 5.6 Interior of the heart

Pot luck

29. What is the function of the chordae tendineae?

_____

_____

_____

30. What is the function of the valves?

_____

_____

_____

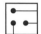 **Labelling**

31. Label the structures indicated in Figure 5.7.

32. Using red arrows, indicate the direction of flow of oxygenated blood through the appropriate vessels and chambers; using blue arrows, do the same for deoxygenated blood.

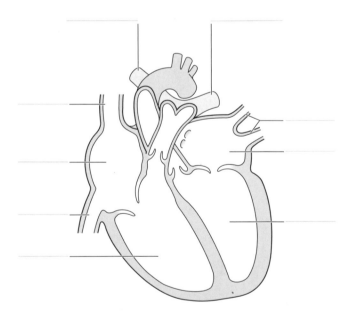

Figure 5.7 Direction of blood flow through the heart

 Matching

33. Put the terms supplied below in the correct order, so that they correctly describe the flow of blood through the pulmonary and systemic circulations, beginning and finishing with the aorta.

Left atrium
Right atrioventricular (tricuspid) valve
Right atrium
Systemic arterial network
Systemic venous network
Left ventricle
Pulmonary valve
Left atrioventricular (mitral) valve
Right ventricle
Pulmonary arteries
Capillaries of body tissues
Aortic valve
Pulmonary veins

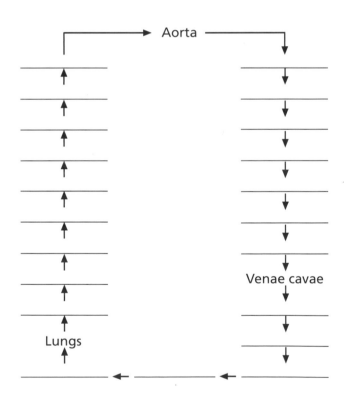

34. Explain why the muscle layer in the left ventricle is thicker than in the right ventricle.

_____

_____

_____

  Matching and colouring

35. In Figure 5.8, identify the left and right sides of the heart, their respective valves, the pulmonary circulation and the systemic circulation and label the capillary beds representing the lungs and the body tissues.

36. Colour the arrows on the diagram representing transport of oxygenated blood red, and arrows showing transport of deoxygenated blood blue.

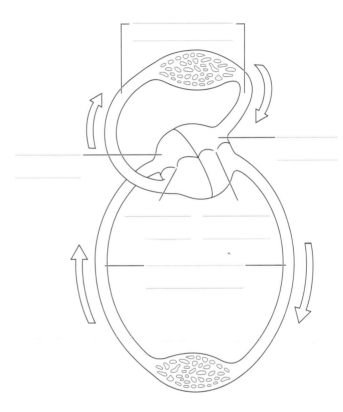

Figure 5.8 Relationship between the pulmonary and systemic circulations

 MCQs

37. How is the heart muscle supplied with oxygen and nutrients? _____.

    a. From the blood that circulates through the heart chambers
    b. By the coronary arteries, which branch from the aorta
    c. By the pulmonary arteries, which also supply the lungs
    d. From the cardiac arteries, which are more extensive on the left side of the heart than the right.

38. How is blood drained from the tissues of the heart? _____.

    a. By venous channels that open into the inferior vena cava
    b. Into the vena cava directly
    c. Mainly into the coronary sinus, which empties into the right atrium
    d. Directly into the pulmonary artery, for oxygenation.

39. What proportion of the cardiac output does the heart itself receive? _____.

   a. 30%   **b.** 20%   **c.** 10%   **d.** 5%.

40. Which chamber of the heart has the largest blood supply? _____.

   a. Right atrium   **b.** Right ventricle   **c.** Left atrium   **d.** Left ventricle.

Colouring and labelling

41. Label the structures indicated on Figure 5.9, which shows the conducting system of the heart, and colour the conducting tissue.

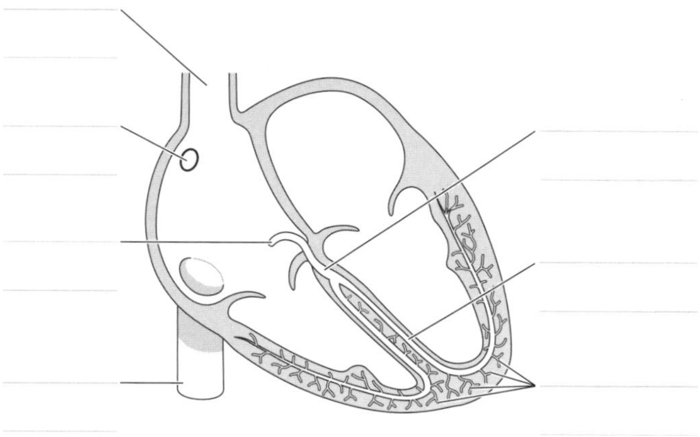

Figure 5.9 Conduction system of the heart

MCQs

42. The heart rate is regulated by the cardiovascular centre, which lies where in the brain? _____.

   a. In the cerebral cortex   **c.** In the medulla oblongata
   b. In the hypothalamus   **d.** In the sympathetic centre.

43. Which of the following lists three effects that will all increase heart rate? _____.

   a. Sympathetic activation; reduced exercise; fear
   b. Adrenaline (epinephrine) release; active exercise; fall in blood pressure
   c. Parasympathetic stimulation; fall in blood pressure; thyroxine release
   d. Rise in blood pressure; adrenaline (epinephrine) release; increased exercise.

44. Which of the following lists three effects that will all decrease heart rate? _____.

   a. Parasympathetic activation; thyroxine release; increase in blood pressure
   b. Adrenaline (epinephrine) release; sympathetic inhibition; reduced exercise
   c. Increase in blood pressure; sympathetic inhibition; sleep
   d. Fear; parasympathetic stimulation; sympathetic inhibition.

45. Which of the following statements is true? _____.

   a. Both the sympathetic and parasympathetic supply to the heart is via the vagus nerve
   b. The sympathetic supply to the heart increases the rate and force of the heartbeat
   c. The sinoatrial node is supplied only by sympathetic nerve fibres
   d. The heart rate slows during parasympathetic activity because of the release of noradrenaline.

Completion

46. Complete the following paragraphs, which describe the cardiac cycle.

Diastole

We will begin this description with the heart in diastole, when the whole heart is _____. During this time, in the upper part of the heart, the atria are _____ and blood is flowing _____. Not only the upper chambers are filling but also the lower ones; because the _____ valves are open, we see that the _____ are filling as well. Although blood is travelling into the lower chambers, at this stage the electrical activity has not reached them yet and so the ventricles are _____. Remember, during this period, the heart muscle is not contracting; both the _____ and the _____ are relaxed.

Atrial systole

The next stage represents atrial systole, or contraction. This is initiated when the _____ fires; its electrical discharge leads to the spread of _____ through the atria. Because of the electrical excitation of the muscle, the atria _____ and this leads to pumping of blood from the _____ into the _____. It is important therefore that the _____ valves are open, to permit blood to flow through. The ventricles fill up; because the _____ and _____ valves are closed, blood cannot yet pass from the heart into the great vessels leaving it.

Ventricular systole

The third stage is ventricular systole. The impulse from the sinoatrial node has passed through the atrioventricular node; inspection of the atria shows that they are _____ after their period of activity; this allows them to rest. However, as far as the lower chambers are concerned, because _____ are spreading through the ventricles, we see that the ventricles _____. So that blood cannot flow in a backwards manner into the atria, the _____ valves are closed. However, for the ventricles to be able to push blood out of the heart, the _____ and _____valves _____. Because of the force generated by the contracting ventricular muscle, blood is pumped from the ventricles into the _____ and the _____.

The cycle is now complete; the heart will enter another period of diastole, allowing the entire organ to rest briefly before the next period of contraction.

? MCQs

47. When the ventricles contract, the atrioventricular valves close, because: _____.

    a. The pressure in the aorta is higher than the pressure in the ventricles
    b. The pressure in the ventricles is higher than the pressure in the atria
    c. The pressure in the atria is higher than the pressure in the pulmonary arteries
    d. The pressure in the aorta is higher than the pressure in the atria.

48. The cardiac valves ensure that flow of blood through the heart is one-way. Where else in the cardiovascular system are there valves doing the same? _____.

    a. Medium sized veins   **b.** Capillaries   **c.** Large veins such as the vena cava   **d.** Arteries.

49. The characteristic sound of the heartbeat through a stethoscope placed over the chest is due to: _____.

    a. Movement of blood through the large vessels leaving and entering the heart
    b. Contraction of the myocardium
    c. Rubbing of the heart against the ribs as it beats
    d. Closing of the valves inside the heart.

50. At which point in the cardiac cycle are the walls of the aorta most stretched? _____.

    a. During atrial systole   **c.** During the first heart sound
    b. When the atrioventricular valves open   **d.** During cardiac diastole.

Labelling

51. Figure 5.10 shows a typical electrocardiograph of one cardiac cycle. Label the individual waves.

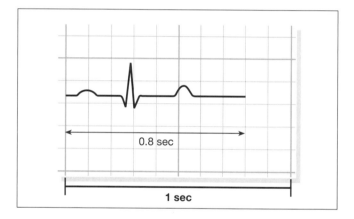

Figure 5.10 The electrocardiogram (ECG)

Matching

52. Match each of the ECG waves named in Figure 5.10 with the corresponding electrical and mechanical events, listed below.

    a. Passage of electrical impulse through the Purkinje fibres: _____.

    b. Atrial systole: _____.

    c. Ventricular relaxation: _____.

    d. Opening of the aortic and pulmonary valves: _____.

    e. Discharge of the sinoatrial node: _____.

    f. Ventricular systole: _____.

    g. Atrial relaxation: _____.

    h. Closure of the atrioventricular valves: _____.

✍ Applying what you know

53. In a man whose heart rate is 80 beats per minute and whose stroke volume is 70 ml, what is the cardiac output? _____.

54. In a woman whose cardiac output is 6 L/min and whose pulse rate is 75 beats per minute, what is the stroke volume? _____.

55. In a man whose cardiac output is 5 L/min and whose stroke volume is 50 ml, what is the heart rate? _____.

？ Pot luck

56. Which of the following would increase stroke volume (assuming no other factor changes to compensate)? Tick all that apply.

 a. Sympathetic stimulation: ____

 b. Increased preload: ____

 c. Increased vagal tone: ____

 d. Increased heart rate: ____

 e. Decreased secretion of adrenaline (epinephrine): ____

 f. Decreased afterload: ____

 g. Increased blood volume: ____

 h. Decreased venous return: ____.

57. Which of the following is associated with increased venous return to the heart (assuming no other factor changes to compensate)? Tick all that apply.

 a. Standing up from a supine position: ____

 b. Decreased blood volume: ____

 c. The skeletal muscle pump: ____

 d. Increased blood pressure: ____

 e. Decreased heart rate: ____

 f. The respiratory pump: ____

 g. Venous congestion: ____

 h. Increased preload: ____.

BLOOD PRESSURE

 MCQs

58. Blood pressure is usually expressed as: _____.

    a Diastolic pressure over systolic pressure   **c.** Systolic pressure over diastolic pressure
    b. Pulse pressure over diastolic pressure   **d.** Diastolic pressure over pulse pressure.

59. Which of the following events can be measured as systolic blood pressure? _____.

    a. Atrial contraction   **b.** Ventricular contraction   **c.** Pulse pressure   **d.** Cardiac diastole.

60. What are the two main factors determining blood pressure? _____.

    a. Cardiac output and peripheral resistance   **c.** Blood volume and pulse pressure
    b. Peripheral resistance and blood volume   **d.** Pulse pressure and cardiac output.

61. Which of the following is associated with the moment-to-moment control of blood pressure? _____.

    a. The renin–angiotensin system   **c.** The baroreceptor reflex
    b. Control of blood volume   **d.** The Hering–Breuer reflex.

 Completion

62. Complete the following paragraphs, which describe the body's control of blood pressure, by scoring out the incorrect options in bold, thus leaving the correct words or phrases.

The baroreceptor reflex is important in the **moment-to-moment/long-term** control of blood pressure. It is controlled by the cardiovascular centre found in the **medulla oblongata/carotid bodies**, and which receives and integrates information from baroreceptors, chemoreceptors and higher centres in the brain. Baroreceptors are receptors sensitive to blood pressure and are found in the **carotid arteries/heart wall/aorta**. A **rise/fall** in blood pressure activates these receptors, which respond by increasing the activity of **parasympathetic/sympathetic** nerve fibres supplying the heart; this **slows the heart down/speeds the heart up** and returns the system towards normal. In addition to this, **sympathetic/parasympathetic** nerve fibres supplying the blood vessels are **activated/inhibited**, which leads to **vasoconstriction/vasodilation**, again returning the system towards normal (note that most blood vessels have little or no **sympathetic/parasympathetic** innervation).

    On the other hand, if the blood pressure **falls/rises**, baroreceptor activity is decreased, and this also triggers compensatory mechanisms. This time, **sympathetic/parasympathetic** activity is increased and this leads to a(n) **reduction/increase** in heart rate; in addition, cardiac contractile force is **increased/reduced**. The blood vessels respond with **vasoconstriction/vasodilation**; this is mainly due to **increased/decreased** activity in **sympathetic/parasympathetic** fibres. These measures lead to a restoration of blood pressure towards normal.

    In addition to the activity of the baroreceptors described above, chemoreceptors in the **carotid bodies/aorta/higher centres of the brain** measure the pH of the blood. Increase in **oxygen/carbon dioxide** content of the blood decreases pH and **stimulates/inhibits** these receptors, leading to an **increase/decrease** in stroke volume and heart rate, and a general **vasoconstriction/vasodilation**; this **increases/decreases** blood pressure. Other control mechanisms include the renin–angiotensin system, which is involved in **long-term/short-term** regulation; activation **increases/decreases** blood volume, thereby **increasing/decreasing** blood pressure.

CIRCULATION OF THE BLOOD

  Colouring and matching

63. On Figure 5.11, indicate the locations of the main pulse points by using different colours in the key.

- ○ Temporal artery
- ○ Carotid artery
- ○ Facial artery
- ○ Femoral artery
- ○ Brachial artery
- ○ Popliteal artery
- ○ Dorsalis pedis artery
- ○ Posterior tibial artery
- ○ Radial artery

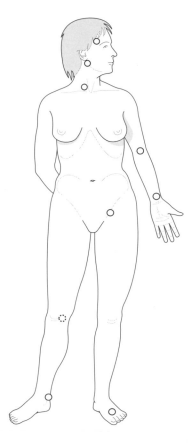

Figure 5.11 Main pulse points

 Completion

64. The following paragraph describes the flow of blood through the pulmonary circulation. Complete it by filling in the blanks.

Blood leaving the right ventricle first enters the _____, which passes upwards close to the aorta and divides into the right _____ and the left _____ at the level of the 5th thoracic vertebra. Each of these branches goes to the corresponding _____, and enters these organs in the area called the _____. Within the tissues, the vessels divide and subdivide, giving a network of many millions of tiny _____, across the walls of which gases exchange. Blood draining these structures then passes through veins of increasing diameter, which finally unite in the _____, which carry the blood back to the _____ atrium of the heart.

Matching

65. The artery leaving the heart and entering the systemic circulation is the aorta, which travels behind the heart, penetrates the diaphragm and descends into the abdomen. Label its main parts and branches using the key choices listed below (L/R = left/right; A = artery).

L. internal iliac A.	Coeliac A.
Inferior mesenteric A.	Ascending aorta
Abdominal aorta	L. common iliac A.
Brachiocephalic A.	R. renal A.
L. subclavian A.	R. subclavian A.
R. common carotid A.	Superior mesenteric A.
Arch of aorta	L. common carotid A.
L. external iliac A.	Thoracic aorta

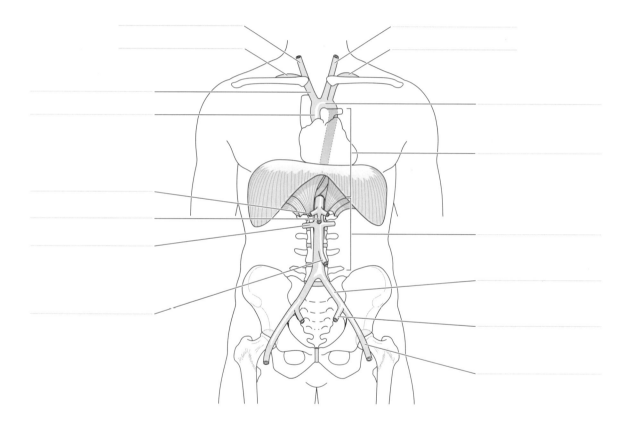

Figure 5.12 The aorta and its main branches

 MCQs

66. Where do the coronary arteries arise? _____.

    a. The aortic arch   **b.** The ascending aorta   **c.** The descending aorta   **d.** The aortic valve.

67. Which artery of those listed below is the most important in the supply to the circulus arteriosus (circle of Willis)? _____.

    a. Internal carotid artery   **c.** Anterior cerebral artery

    b. External carotid artery   **d.** Anterior communicating artery.

68. Which artery is important in supplying the superficial tissues of the head and neck? _____.

    a. Internal carotid artery   **c.** Anterior cerebral artery

    b. External carotid artery   **d.** Anterior communicating artery.

69. From which artery does the vertebral artery arise? _____.

    a. Aorta   **b.** Internal carotid artery   **c.** Subclavian artery   **d.** Brachiocephalic artery.

70. Which is the major vein draining the tissues of the head and upper body? _____.

    a. Anterior jugular vein   **b.** Superior vena cava   **c.** Inferior vena cava   **d.** Internal jugular vein.

71. The right and left brachiocephalic veins unite to form the: _____.

    a. Brachial vein   **b.** Internal jugular vein   **c.** Superior vena cava   **d.** Subclavian vein.

Labelling

72. Figure 5.13 shows the circulus arteriosus (circle of Willis), which is important in supplying most of the brain. Label the arteries indicated.

73. Venous blood from deep areas of the brain is collected in channels called sinuses, which empty ultimately into the internal jugular veins. Figure 5.14 shows the main venous sinuses of the left side of the brain (remember a mirror image will also exist on the right hand side). Label the sinuses indicated.

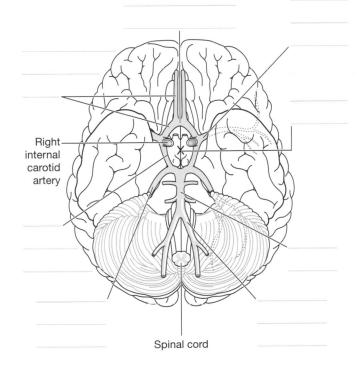

Right internal carotid artery

Spinal cord

Figure 5.13 The circulus arteriosus (circle of Willis)

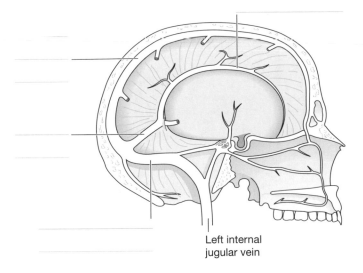

Left internal jugular vein

Figure 5.14 Venous sinuses of the brain

Labelling and colouring

74. Figures 5.15 and 5.16 show the main arteries and veins of the limbs. Label the vessels shown, and colour the arteries in red and the veins in blue.

Figure 5.15 Aorta and main arteries

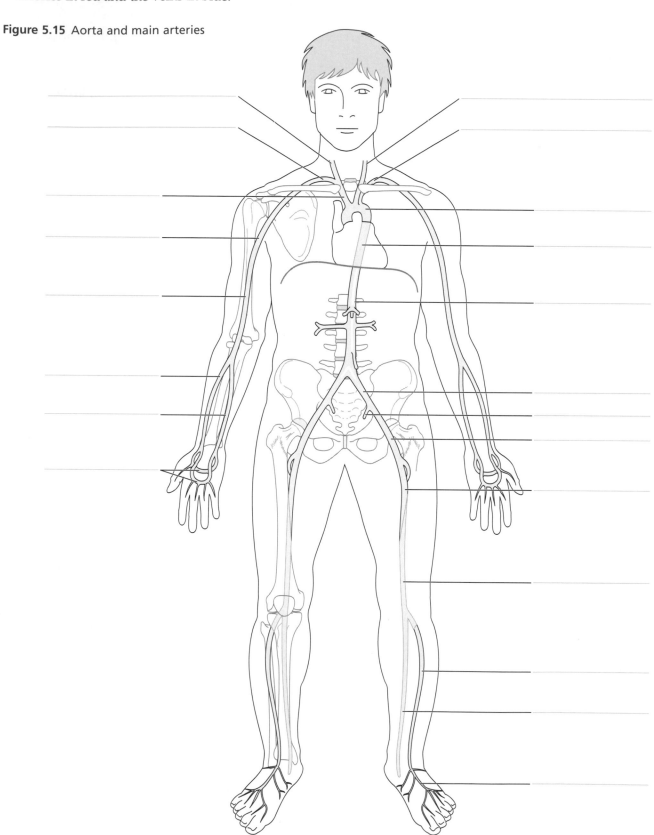

Figure 5.16 Venae cavae and main veins

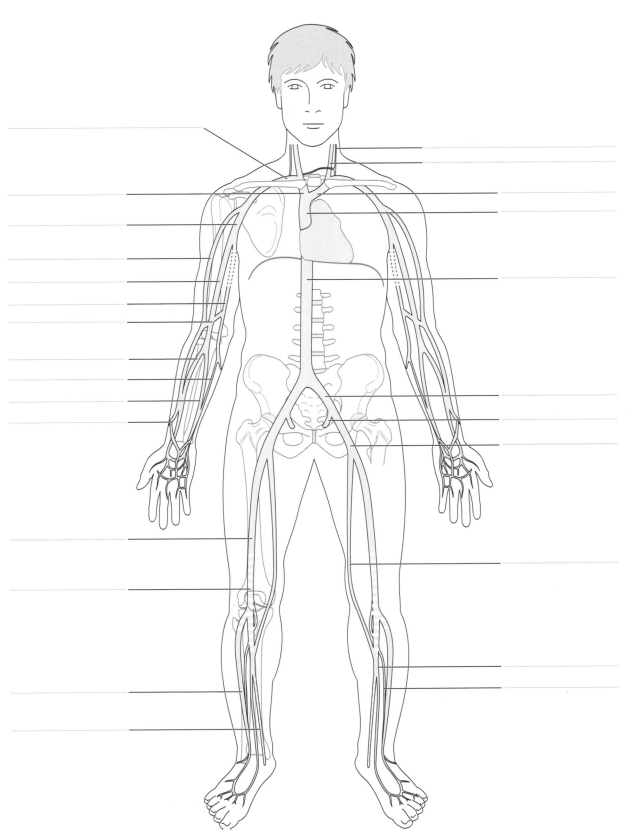

? MCQs

75. Which artery links the axillary artery with the radial artery? _____.

    a. Ulnar artery   **b.** Subclavian artery   **c.** Brachial artery   **d.** Palmar arteries.

76. Many of the veins draining the upper limb are named for, and run alongside, the corresponding artery. Which of the following does not? _____.

    a. Palmar venous arch **b.** Metacarpal vein   **c.** Digital vein   **d.** Median cubital vein.

77. Into which vein does the cephalic vein empty? _____.

    a. Basilic vein   **b.** Axillary vein   **c.** Subclavian vein   **d.** Brachial vein.

78. The inferior vena cava is formed by the union of which vessels? _____.

    a. Left and right common iliac veins   **c.** Femoral vein and saphenous vein
    b. Internal and external iliac veins   **d.** Common iliac vein and femoral vein.

↰↳ Matching

79. Trace the flow of blood from the heart through the leg by putting the vessels listed below in the correct order, starting with the aorta and finishing with the inferior vena cava.

Femoral vein
Anterior tibial vein
Dorsalis pedis artery
Femoral artery
Digital arteries
External iliac vein
Common iliac artery
Popliteal vein
Dorsal venous arch
Popliteal artery
Common iliac vein
Anterior tibial artery

Aorta
↓
_____
↓
External iliac artery
↓
_____
↓
_____
↓
_____
↓
_____
↓
_____

Inferior vena cava
↑
_____
↑
_____
↑
_____
↑
_____
↑
_____
↑
Digital veins

? MCQs

80. Which of the following do not arise directly from the thoracic aorta? _____.

    a. Oesophageal arteries   **b.** Bronchial arteries   **c.** Intercostal arteries   **d.** Mesenteric arteries.

81. At which point does the thoracic aorta become the abdominal aorta (choose all that apply)? _____.

    a. Where the aortic arch terminates   **c.** Where the aorta passes through the diaphragm
    b. At the level of the 12th thoracic vertebra   **d.** At the division of the aorta into the two common iliac arteries.

82. Which of the following branches of the abdominal aorta is unpaired? _____.

    a. Phrenic artery   **b.** Renal artery   **c.** Coeliac artery   **d.** Ovarian artery.

83. The hepatic artery is an unpaired artery and supplies which of the following organs, either all or in part (choose all that apply)? _____.

    a. Liver   **b.** Stomach   **c.** Pancreas   **d.** Gall bladder.

84. Most of the venous drainage in the abdomen is by veins named for their corresponding arteries, but an important exception is the portal vein that links which two sets of abdominal organs? _____.

    a. The liver and the kidneys   **c.** The liver and the intestines
    b. The kidneys and the intestines   **d.** The liver and the gall bladder.

85. What unusual arrangement of blood vessels is associated with the portal circulation? _____.

    a. Capillaries in the liver drain directly into the portal vein
    b. Blood passes through two sets of capillaries before returning to the venous circulation
    c. The portal vein is formed from the union of several other veins
    d. The portal vein links the arterial and venous circulations without an intervening capillary bed.

86. The physiological function of the portal circulation is to: _____.

    a. Slow blood flow through the liver sinusoids so that the blood can be appropriately modified
    b. Supply the liver cells with nutrients and oxygen
    c. Regulate the concentrations of blood constituents in blood coming from the intestines
    d. Increase the blood supply to the liver, which is metabolically very active.

87. The cystic vein drains blood from the: _____.

    a. Urinary bladder   **b.** Gall bladder   **c.** Pancreas   **d.** Kidneys.

Matching, colouring and labelling

88. On Figure 5.17, label the structures indicated using the labels provided.

Abdominal aorta	Lung
Inferior vena cava	Ductus arteriosus
Right ventricle	Aortic arch
Foramen ovale	Common iliac artery
Hepatic portal vein	Liver
Umbilicus	Right atrium
Placenta	Ductus venosus
Superior vena cava	Umbilical cord
Pulmonary artery	Pulmonary veins
Umbilical vein	Umbilical arteries

89. On Figure 5.17, insert arrows on the umbilical
    arteries and vein, pulmonary arteries and veins,
    right and left sides of the heart, aorta, foramen
    ovale and ductus arteriosus to show direction of
    blood flow through the foetal circulation.

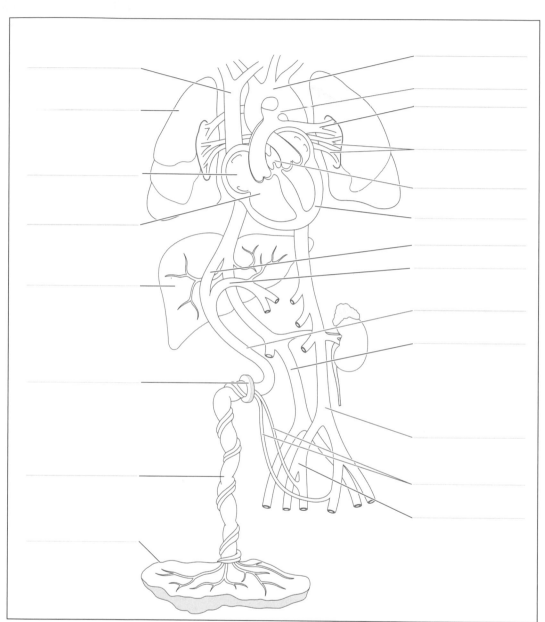

Figure 5.17
The foetal circulation.

 Pot luck

90. List the functions of the placenta.

    • _____

    • _____

    • _____.

6 The lymphatic system

The lymphatic system consists of a network of lymphatic vessels, the fluid that flows through them and various specialized organs and tissues. Its main functions are in tissue drainage and in the production and maintenance of immune cells.

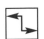   **Matching, colouring and labelling**

1. Figure 6.1 shows the main structures of the lymphatic system. Label the structures indicated using the key choices listed.

Key choices:

Inguinal nodes

Lymphatic vessels

Thymus gland

Red bone marrow

Palatine tonsil

Thoracic duct (twice)

Spleen

Aggregated lymph follicles (Peyer's patches)

Submandibular nodes

Cisterna chyli

Intestinal nodes

Axillary nodes

Right lymphatic duct

2. On Figure 6.1, colour the spleen, red bone marrow of the right femur and the thymus gland different colours, using the key below.

```
○ Spleen
○ Thymus gland
○ Red bone marrow
```

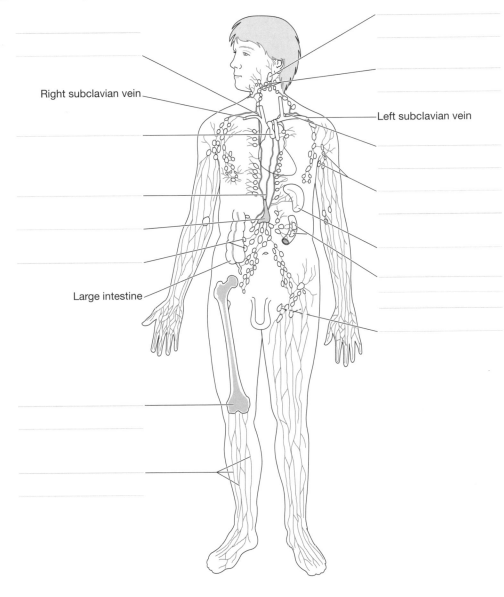

Figure 6.1 The lymphatic system

3. List the three main functions of the lymphatic system:

• _____

• _____

• _____.

LYMPH

 MCQs

4. Which important constituent of plasma is absent from lymph? _____.

    a. Glucose   **b.** Plasma proteins   **c.** Hormones   **d.** Antibodies.

5. What is the difference between lymph and interstitial fluid? _____.

    a. Lymph contains white blood cells and interstitial fluid does not
    b. Nothing – the two terms are interchangeable
    c. Interstitial fluid bathes the cells and lymph is found in the lymphatic vessels
    d. Lymph becomes interstitial fluid when it returns to the bloodstream.

6. Which nutrient is absorbed into the lymphatic vessels of the small intestine? _____.

    a. Glucose   **b.** Amino acids   **c.** Vitamins   **d.** Fats.

7. Lymphocytes, which circulate in the lymph, are produced in the: _____.

    a. Spleen   **b.** Thymus gland   **c.** Red bone marrow   **d.** Cisterna chyli.

LYMPHATIC VESSELS

Completion

8. The following paragraph describes lymphatic vessels. Complete it by scoring out the incorrect options in bold, leaving the correct option(s).

The smallest lymphatic vessels are called **ducts/venules/capillaries**. One significant difference between them and the smallest blood vessels is that they **are only one cell thick/have permeable walls/originate in the tissues**; their function is to drain the lymph, containing **red blood cells/white blood cells/platelets**, away from the interstitial spaces. Most tissues have a network of these tiny vessels, but one notable exception is **bone tissue/muscle tissue/fatty tissue**. The individual tiny vessels join up to form larger ones, which now contain **two/three/four** layers of tissue in their walls, similar to veins in the cardiovascular system. The inner lining, the **endothelial/fibrous/muscular** layer, covers the valves, which **filter the lymph/store the lymph/regulate flow of lymph**. Unlike the cardiovascular system, there is no organ acting as a pump to push lymph through the vessels, but forward pressure is applied to the lymph by various mechanisms, including **movement of the valves pushing lymph onward/squeezing of the vessels by external structures like skeletal muscle/intrinsic contractility of the smooth muscle of lymphatic vessel walls**. As vessels progressively unite and become wider and wider, eventually they empty into the biggest lymph vessels of all, the **thoracic duct and the right lymphatic duct/subclavian duct and the right lymphatic duct/thoracic duct and subclavian duct**. The first one of these drains the **left side of the body/right side of the body above the diaphragm/lower limbs and pelvic area**. The second drains the **upper body above the pelvis/right side of the body/lower part of the body and the upper left side above the diaphragm**.

LYMPHATIC ORGANS AND TISSUES

  ### Labelling and colouring

9. Figure 6.2 shows the internal structure of a lymph node. Label the structures indicated and colour the capsule and associated trabeculae.

10. On Figure 6.2, insert arrows to show which way lymph will flow through this lymph node.

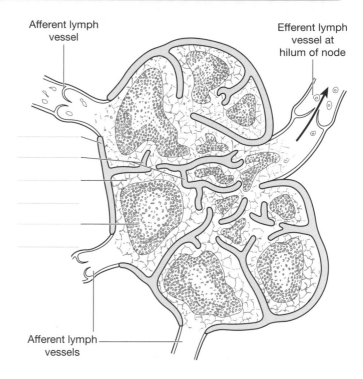

Afferent lymph vessel

Efferent lymph vessel at hilum of node

Afferent lymph vessels

Figure 6.2 Section of a lymph node

 ### MCQs

11. What are the main types of tissue that make up a lymph node? _____.

   a. Blood and lymphatic vessels
   b. Capsular tissue and its associated trabeculae
   c. Reticular and lymphatic tissue
   d. Lymphatic vessels in connective tissue.

12. Which important protective cells are found within lymph nodes? _____.

   a. Lymphocytes and macrophages
   b. Neutrophils and antibodies
   c. Red blood cells and monocytes
   d. Eosinophils and granulocytes.

13. Which of the following statements is true concerning the structure of a lymph node? ____.

   a. They have no blood supply but receive their nutrients and oxygen from the lymph that passes through
   b. Each node has several efferent vessels but only one afferent vessel
   c. The cisterna chyli is the biggest lymph node in the body
   d. Each node has a concave surface called the hilum where various vessels enter and leave the node.

14. Which is the main group of nodes draining the breast? _____.

   a. The mammary nodes
   b. The axillary nodes
   c. The inguinal nodes
   d. The cervical nodes.

 ### Definition

15. Define the term phagocytosis: _____

   _____.

? Pot luck

16. The function of lymph nodes is to filter and clean lymph. List at least four types of particulate matter that are removed from the lymph:

- _____
- _____

- _____
- _____ .

17. What happens to organic materials phagocytosed in the lymph nodes?

_____

18. What happens to inorganic materials phagocytosed in the lymph nodes?

_____

_____

Matching

19. For each of the following key choices, decide whether it applies to the lymph nodes, the spleen or the thymus, and complete Table 6.1.

Key choices:

T-lymphocytes mature here
Bean-shaped
Largest lymphatic organ
Site of multiplication of activated lymphocytes
Stores blood
Made up of two narrow lobes
Red blood cells destroyed here
Distributed throughout lymphatic system
Maximum weight usually 30–40 g

Lies immediately below the diaphragm
At its maximum size in puberty
Filters lymph
Oval in shape
Lies immediately behind the sternum
Size from pinhead to almond size
Secretes the hormone thymosin
Synthesizes red blood cells in the fetus
Phagocytoses cellular debris

Spleen	Thymus	Lymph node

Table 6.1 Characteristics of lymph nodes, spleen and thymus

MCQs

20. Mucosa-associated lymphoid tissue (MALT): _____

    a. is enclosed within a protective capsule
    b. filters lymph
    c. contains T- and B-lymphocytes
    d. is found only in the gastrointestinal tract.

21. Tonsils are made up of lymphatic tissue and: _____

    a. do not filter lymph
    b. produce saliva
    c. are well supplied with afferent lymphatic vessels
    d. are found in a ring around the larynx.

22. Aggregated lymph follicles (Peyer's patches) are found in the: _____

    a. throat
    b. lungs
    c. gastrointestinal tract
    d. lymph nodes.

23. Thymosin: _____

    a. is produced by the thyroid gland
    b. is responsible for maturation of the thymus
    c. is an essential cofactor in antibody production
    d. levels increase with age.

7 The nervous system

The nervous system detects and quickly responds to changes inside and outside the body. Together with the endocrine system, it controls important aspects of body function. Responses to changes in the internal environment maintain homeostasis and regulate our involuntary functions. Responses to changes in the external environment maintain posture and other voluntary activities.

The nervous system consists of the brain, spinal cord and peripheral nerves organized in a way that enables rapid communication between different parts of the body. This chapter is designed to help you learn about the structure and functions of the nervous system and its components.

 ## Matching and labelling

1. Name the two main parts of the central nervous system:

   • _____

   • _____

2. Label the sensory and motor neurones on Figure 7.1.

3. Insert the key choices beside the bullet points on Figure 7.1 showing their relationships to the nervous system.

Key choices:
Chemoreceptors   Sight   Smooth muscle   Taste   Skeletal muscle   Osmoreceptors
Glands   Hearing   Baroreceptors   Cardiac muscle Smell

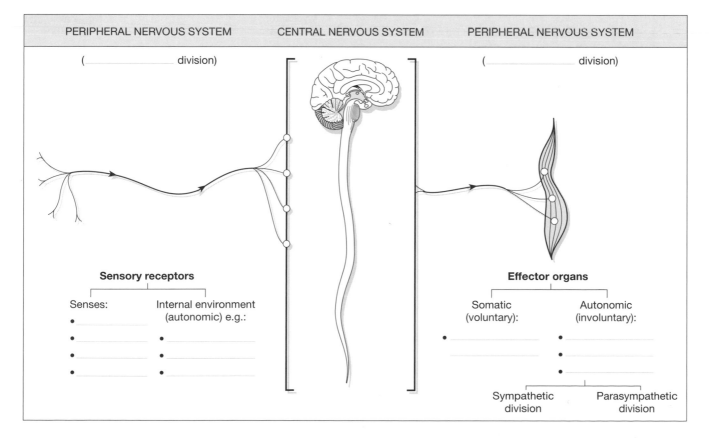

Figure 7.1 Functional components of the nervous system

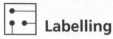 **Labelling**

4. Label the parts of the neurone indicated in Figure 7.2.

5. Draw an arrow beside a neurone in Figure 7.2 to show the direction of impulse conduction.

6. Outline the main difference between the structure of myelinated and non-myelinated neurones.

_____

_____

_____

_____

_____.

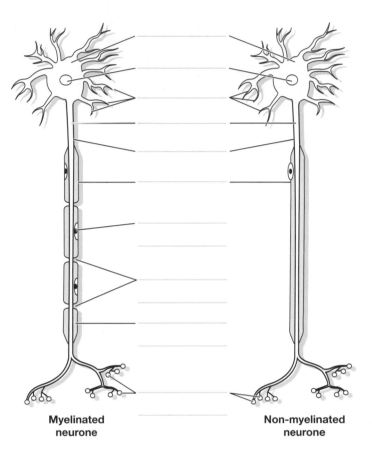

Myelinated neurone   **Non-myelinated neurone**

Figure 7.2 The structure of neurones

 Matching

7. Match the correct key choice with the appropriate statement. (Take care, as you will not need all the key choices.)

Key choices:

Tracts	Nuclei	Afferent
Cell bodies	Neurones	Conductive
Axons	Ganglia	Efferent

a. Form the grey matter of the nervous system: _____

b. Groups of cell bodies in the central nervous system: _____

c. Groups of axons found deep in the brain and at the periphery of the spinal cord: _____

d. Nerve fibres that carry impulses towards the central nervous system: _____

e. Form the white matter of the nervous system: _____

f. Groups of cell bodies in the peripheral nervous system: _____

g. Nerve fibres that carry impulses from the central nervous system: _____.

Completion

8. Fill in the blanks in the paragraph below to describe the events that occur during conduction of nerve impulses.

Transmission of the _____, or impulse, is due to movement of _____ across the nerve cell membrane. In the resting state the nerve cell membrane is _____ due to differences in the concentrations of ions across the plasma membrane. This means that there is a different electrical charge on each side of the membrane, which is called the resting _____. At rest the charge outside the cell is _____ and inside it is _____. The principal ions involved are _____ and _____. In the resting state there is a continual tendency for these ions to diffuse down their _____. During the action potential, sodium ions flood _____ the neurone causing _____. This is followed by _____ when potassium ions move _____ the neurone. In myelinated neurones the insulating properties of the _____ prevent the movement of ions across the membrane where this is present. In these neurones, impulses pass from one _____ to the next and transmission is called _____. In unmyelinated fibres, nerve impulses are conducted by the process called _____. Impulse conduction is faster when the mechanism of transmission is _____ than when it is _____. The diameter of the neurone also affects the rate of impulse conduction: the _____ the diameter, the faster the conduction.

Colouring, matching and labelling

9. Colour and match the following on each part of Figure 7.3:

○ Presynaptic neurone
○ Postsynaptic neurone

10. Label the structures indicated on Figure 7.3.

11. Add arrows showing the direction of impulse transmission in the neurones shown on the main part of Figure 7.3.

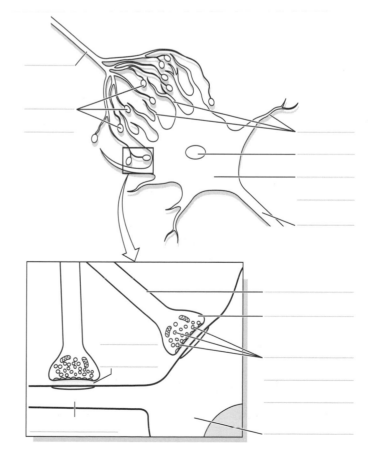

Figure 7.3 Diagram of a synapse

Completion

12. Fill in the blanks to complete the paragraph below, describing the transmission of an impulse from one neurone to the next.

The region where a nerve impulse passes from one neurone to another is called the _____. The distal end

of the presynaptic neurone breaks up into minute branches known as _____. These are in close

proximity to the dendrites and cell bodies of the _____. The space between them is the

_____. In the ends of the presynaptic neurones are spherical structures called _____

containing chemicals known as the _____. When the action potential depolarizes the presynaptic

membrane, the chemicals in the membrane-bound packages are released into the synaptic cleft by the process of

_____. The chemicals released then move across the synaptic cleft by _____. They act on

specific areas of the postsynaptic membrane called _____ causing _____.

CENTRAL NERVOUS SYSTEM

? **Pot luck**

13. This exercise considers characteristics of the different types of non-excitable cells found in the central nervous system. For each statement below, identify which of the following it refers to:

| Astrocytes | Microglia | Oligodendrocytes | Ependymal cells |

a. The main supporting tissue of the central nervous system is formed by: _____.

b. These cells provide protection when they become phagocytic in areas of inflammation:

_____.

c. The cells found along the length of myelinated nerve fibres are: _____.

d. The star-shaped supporting cells are: _____.

e. The lining of the ventricles of the brain and the central canal of the spinal cord is formed by:

_____.

f. These cells form and maintain myelin: _____.

g. Found in large numbers around blood vessels, with their foot processes forming the blood–brain barrier,

these cells are: _____.

14. Outline the function of the blood–brain barrier.

_____

_____.

 Completion

15. Complete Table 7.1 by ticking the appropriate columns(s) for each statement about the meninges.

	Dura mater	Arachnoid mater	Pia mater
Consists of two layers of fibrous tissue			
Consists of fine connective tissue			
A delicate serous membrane			
The subdural space lies between these two layers			
Surrounds the venous sinuses			
The subarachnoid space separates these two layers			
Forms the filum terminale			
CSF is found in the space between these two layers			
Equivalent to the periosteum of other bones			

Table 7.1 Characteristics of the meninges

Labelling

16. Label the meninges and other structures indicated on Figure 7.4.

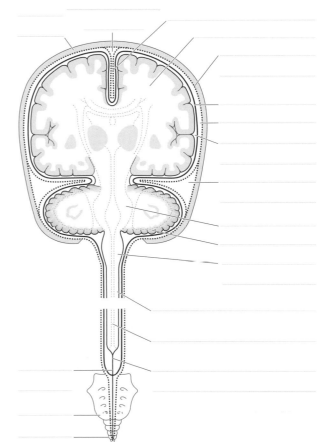

Figure 7.4 The meninges covering the brain and spinal cord

Colouring and labelling

17. Colour the ventricular system of the brain.

18. Label the components of the ventricular system identified in Figure 7.5.

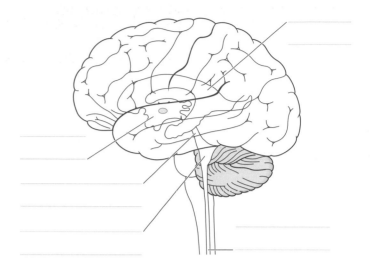

Figure 7.5 The positions of the ventricles in the brain viewed from the left side

? MCQs

19. Which of the following is necessary for the secretion of cerebrospinal fluid (choose all that apply)? _____.

    a. Arachnoid villi   **b.** Choroid plexuses   **c.** Third ventricle   **d.** Fourth ventricle.

20. CSF circulation is aided by (choose all that apply): _____.

    a. Breathing   **b.** Pulsing blood vessels   **c.** A pump   **d.** Changes in posture.

21. CSF normally contains: _____.

    a. Glucose, albumin, red blood cells, white blood cells   **c.** Globulin, red blood cells, glucose, albumin
    b. White blood cells, red blood cells, albumin, globulin   **d.** Albumin, globulin, white blood cells, glucose.

22. CSF passes into the blood through the: _____.

    a. Central canal   **b.** Arachnoid villi   **c.** Corpus callosum   **d.** Choroid plexuses.

 ## ? Pot luck

23. List four functions of CSF:

- _____

- _____

- _____

- _____.

BRAIN

  Colouring, matching and labelling

24. Colour, match and label the following parts of the
central nervous system on Figure 7.6:

○ Cerebrum
○ Cerebellum
○ Medulla oblongata
○ Midbrain
○ Pons
○ Spinal cord

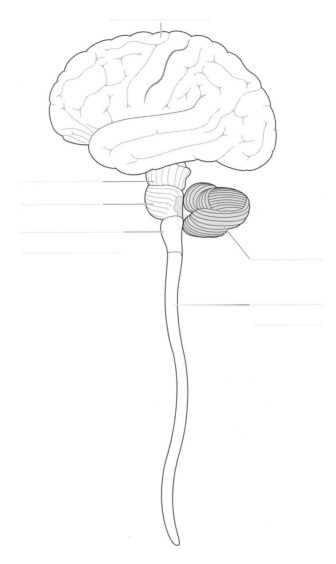

Figure 7.6 The parts of the central nervous system

 Completion

25. Complete the blanks to describe the structure of the cerebrum.

This is the largest part of the brain and is divided into left and right _____. Deep inside, the

two parts are connected by the _____, which consists of _____ matter. The superficial layer of the

cerebrum is known as the _____ and consists of nerve _____ or _____ matter. The

deeper layer consists of nerve _____ and is _____ in colour. The cerebral cortex has many furrows and

folds that vary in depth. The exposed areas are the convolutions or _____ and they are separated by

_____, also known as _____. These convolutions increase the _____ of the cerebrum.

Colouring and matching

26. Colour the structures listed below, matching them with those on Figure 7.7.

- ○ Corpus callosum
- ○ Basal ganglia
- ○ Thalamus
- ○ Internal capsule
- ○ Cerebral cortex
- ○ Hypothalamus

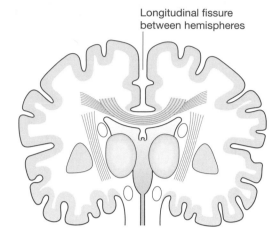

Longitudinal fissure between hemispheres

Figure 7.7 A section of the cerebrum showing some connecting nerve fibres

27. List the three main functions of the cerebrum:

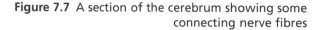

- _____
- _____
- _____ .

  Colouring, matching and labelling

28. Colour, match and label the functional areas of the cerebrum listed below with those identified in Figure 7.8:

- ○ Taste area
- ○ Somatosensory area
- ○ Primary motor area
- ○ Frontal area
- ○ Sensory speech (Wernicke's) area
- ○ Auditory area
- ○ Motor speech (Broca's) area
- ○ Premotor area
- ○ Visual area

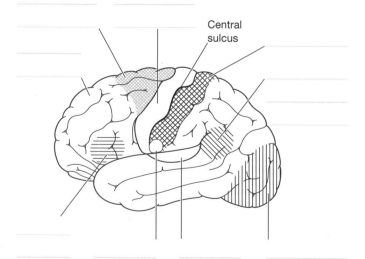

Central sulcus

Figure 7.8 The cerebrum showing the functional areas

Completion

29. The following paragraphs describe aspects of the motor areas of the cerebrum. Cross out the wrong options so that it reads correctly.

The primary motor area lies in the **parietal/temporal/frontal** lobe immediately anterior to the **central/lateral/parieto-occipital** sulcus. The cell bodies are **oval/pyramid-shaped/hexagonal** and stimulation leads to contraction of **smooth/skeletal/cardiac** muscle. Their nerve fibres pass downwards through the **thalamus/internal capsule/hypothalamus** to the **midbrain/cerebellum/medulla** where they cross to the opposite side then descend in the spinal cord. These neurones are the upper motor neurones. They synapse with the lower motor neurones in the **spinal cord/medulla/cerebellum** and lower motor neurones terminate at a **neuromuscular junction/ synapse/sensory receptor**. This means that the motor area of the right hemisphere controls skeletal muscle movement on **the left/the right/both sides(s)** of the body.

In the motor area of the cerebrum, body areas are represented **in mirror image/the right way up/upside down** and the proportion of the cerebral cortex that represents a particular part of the body reflects its **size/complexity of movement/distance from the brain.**

Broca's area lies in the **parietal/temporal/frontal** lobe and controls the movements needed for **swallowing/writing/speech**. The right hemisphere is dominant in **left-handed/ambidextrous/right-handed** people.

The frontal area is situated in the **parietal/frontal/temporal** lobe and is thought to be involved in one's **body clock/feelings of hunger/character.**

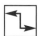 ## Matching

30. Match the statements below with the sensory areas of the cerebrum listed (you will need some sensory areas more than once):

> Olfactory area
> Gustatory area
> Visual area
> Auditory area
> Sensory speech area

a. The left side is dominant in right-handed people: _____.

b. The centre for perception of taste: _____.

c. Receives impulses from the 8th cranial nerves: _____.

d. The centre for the perception of smell: _____.

e. Receives impulses from the 2nd cranial nerves: _____.

f. Receives impulses from the 1st cranial nerves: _____.

g. The centre for hearing: _____.

h. Sensory nerves are activated by chemicals in solution: _____.

i. The most posterior sensory area of the brain: _____.

j. Situated in the temporal lobe: _____.

k. The centre for sight: _____.

? MCQs

31. Which of the following is not part of the brainstem? _____.

    a. Midbrain   **b.** Pons   **c.** Cerebellum   **d.** Medulla.

32. The hypothalamus is involved in control of (choose all that apply): _____.

    a. The autonomic nervous system   **c.** Blood glucose levels
    b. Body temperature   **d.** Thirst and water balance.

33. Important masses of grey matter in the cerebrum include the (choose all that apply): _____.

    a. Basal ganglia   **b.** Pons   **c.** Thalamus   **d.** Reticular formation.

34. The vital centres are found within the: _____.

    a. Midbrain   **b.** Pons   **c.** Cerebellum   **d.** Medulla.

35. The vital centres include the (choose all that apply): _____.

    a. Respiratory centre   **b.** Sleep centre   **c.** Basal ganglia   **d.** Vomiting centre.

36. The reticular formation: _____.

    a. Is a collection of neurones in the cerebellum   **c.** Is involved in control of respiration
    b. Filters sensory information to the cerebrum   **d.** Contains several reflex centres.

37. Which of the following is *not* a function of the cerebellum? _____.

    a. Maintaining balance   **c.** Coordinating movement
    b. Maintaining posture   **d.** Associating sensations and emotions.

38. Proprioceptor impulses come from the: _____.

    a. Brain   **b.** Skin   **c.** Joints   **d.** Eyes.

SPINAL CORD

? Pot luck

39. What is a lumbar puncture? _____

_____

40. Identify the points of origin and destination of the following tracts:

    a. Spinothalamic: origin _____; destination _____.

    b. Corticospinal: origin _____; destination _____.

Completion

41. Tick the appropriate boxes in Table 7.2 to indicate whether each statement relates to either sensory or motor pathways that travel through the spinal cord.

	Motor pathways	Sensory pathways
Impulses travel towards the brain		
The extrapyramidal tracts are an example of these		
Consist of two neurones		
Contain afferent tracts		
Their fibres pass through the internal capsule		
Impulses from proprioceptors travel via these pathways		
Are involved in fine movements		
Are involved in movement of skeletal muscles		
Impulses follow activation of receptors in the skin		
Impulses travel away from the brain		
May consist of either two or three neurones		

Table 7.2 Characteristics of the motor and sensory pathways of the spinal cord

 Completion and labelling

42. On Figure 7.10, draw in:

- the skin around the sensory nerve endings
- the skeletal muscle fibres with motor end-plates.

43. Label the structures identified on Figure 7.9.

44. Draw arrows indicating the direction of the nerve impulses in a reflex arc on Figure 7.9.

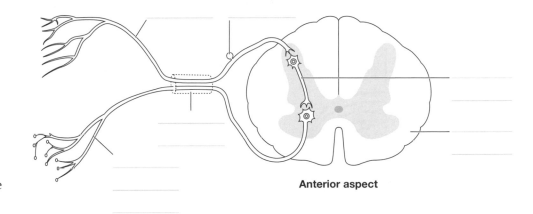

Anterior aspect

Figure 7.9 A simple reflex arc involving one side only

PERIPHERAL NERVOUS SYSTEM

✎ Completion

45. Complete the following paragraph, describing the peripheral nervous system, by filling in the blanks.

Within the peripheral nervous system there are _____ pairs of spinal nerves and _____ pairs of cranial nerves. These nerves are composed of _____ nerve fibres conveying afferent impulses to _____ from _____ organs, or _____ nerve fibres that transmit efferent impulses from _____ to _____ organs. Some nerves, known as _____ nerves contain both types of fibres.

46. Explain the function of a nerve plexus.

_____

_____

⠿ Labelling

47. Name the plexuses and other structures shown on Figure 7.10.

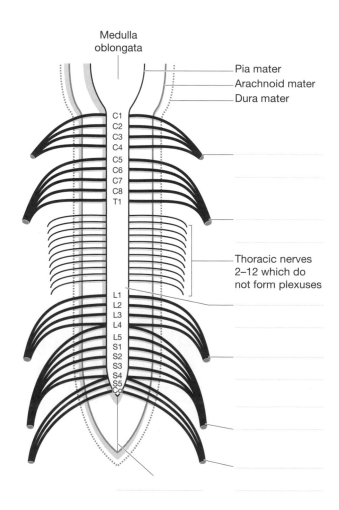

Medulla oblongata

Pia mater
Arachnoid mater
Dura mater

C1
C2
C3
C4
C5
C6
C7
C8
T1

Thoracic nerves 2–12 which do not form plexuses

L1
L2
L3
L4
L5
S1
S2
S3
S4
S5
Co

Figure 7.10 The meninges covering the spinal cord, spinal nerves and the plexuses they form

⠿ ↰ Labelling and matching

48. Label and match the following nerves of the arm shown on the anterior view of Figure 7.11:

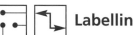

Ulnar	Radial	Median

49. Label and match the following nerves of the arm shown on the posterior view of Figure 7.11:

Ulnar (× 2 labels)	Radial (× 2 labels)	Axillary

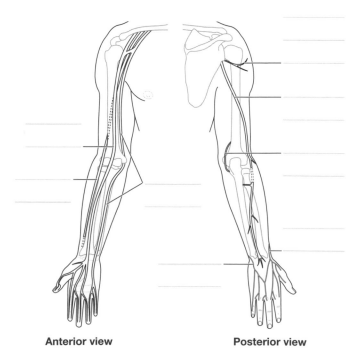

Anterior view   **Posterior view**

Figure 7.11 The main nerves of the arm

Labelling and matching

50. Label and match the following nerves of the leg shown on the anterior view of Figure 7.12:

> Sural
> Femoral
> Obturator
> Common peroneal
> Saphenous
> Deep peroneal
> Superficial peroneal
> Lateral cutaneous nerve of thigh

51. Label and match the following nerves of the leg shown on the posterior view of Figure 7.12:

> Common peroneal
> Posterior cutaneous nerve of thigh
> Sural
> Sciatic
> Tibial (× 2 labels)

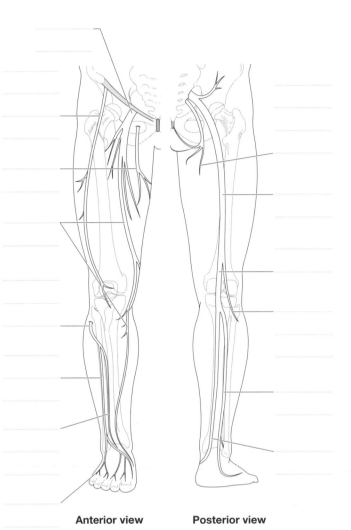

Anterior view   **Posterior view**

Figure 7.12 The main nerves of the leg

 Pot luck

52. Name the nerves that supply the:

   a. Intercostal muscles: _____

   b. Diaphragm: _____

   c. Hamstrings: _____

   d. External anal sphincter: _____

   e. External urethral sphincter: _____.

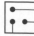 ## Colouring and labelling

53. Identify the parts of the central nervous system indicated on the left side of Figure 7.13.

54. Colour the cranial nerves and their associated structures on Figure 7.13.

55. Name the numbered cranial nerves on the right side of Figure 7.13.

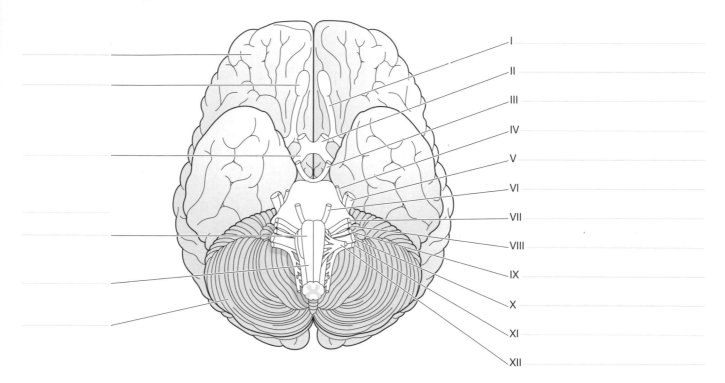

Figure 7.13 The inferior surface of the brain showing the cranial nerves

 ## Completion

56. Insert the names and functions of the cranial nerves in the appropriate boxes in Table 7.3.

57. Identify the type of each cranial nerve (sensory, motor or mixed) to complete Table 7.3.

Table 7.3 The cranial nerves and their functions

Number	Name	Function	Type
I			
II			
III			
IV			
V			
VI			
VII			
VIII			
IX			
X			
XI			
XII			

? MCQs

58. Which of the following are branches of the trigeminal nerve (choose all that apply)? _____.

   a. Facial nerve   **b.** Ophthalmic nerve   **c.** Maxillary nerve   **d.** Mandibular nerve.

59. The vestibulocochlear nerve consists of which two sensory parts? _____.

   a. Vestibular   **b.** Aural   **c.** Oral   **d.** Cochlear.

60. The cranial nerves involved in the swallowing and gag reflexes are the: _____.

   a. Vagus   **b.** Facial   **c.** Glossopharyngeal   **d.** Abducent.

61. The cranial nerves with the most extensive distribution are the: _____.

   a. Trigeminal   **b.** Vagus   **c .** Glossopharyngeal   **d.** Facial.

62. Which nerves cause constriction of the pupils? _____.

   a. Optic   **b.** Oculomotor   **c.** Trochlear   **d.** Abducent.

63. Which cranial nerves supply the accessory muscles of respiration? _____.

   a. Accessory   **b.** Abducent   **c.** Vagus   **d.** Intercostal.

AUTONOMIC NERVOUS SYSTEM

? Pot luck

64. Name the effector organs of the autonomic nervous system:

   • _____

   • _____

   • _____.

65. List the two divisions of the autonomic nervous system:

   • _____

   • _____.

66. Decide whether each of the following statements is TRUE or FALSE:

   a. The sympathetic nervous system is sometimes referred to as the craniosacral outflow: _____

   b. The parasympathetic nervous system is associated with fight or flight responses: _____

   c. The parasympathetic nervous system has a preganglionic and a postganglionic neurone: _____

   d. The neurotransmitter at the sympathetic ganglia is noradrenaline: _____

   e. The neurotransmitter at the parasympathetic ganglionic synapse is acetylcholine: _____

   f. Stimulation of the parasympathetic nervous system results in release of adrenaline from the adrenal glands: _____

   g. There is no sympathetic nerve supply to sweat glands: _____

   h. In the parasympathetic nervous system, the preganglionic fibre is longer than the postganglionic fibre: _____.

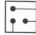 **Colouring and labelling**

67. Draw in lines to represent the postganglionic sympathetic fibres on Figure 7.14.

68. Label the three prevertebral ganglia shown on Figure 7.14.

69. Colour and name the structures supplied by the sympathetic nervous system shown in Figure 7.14.

70. Complete Figure 7.14 by inserting the effects of sympathetic stimulation in the right-hand column.

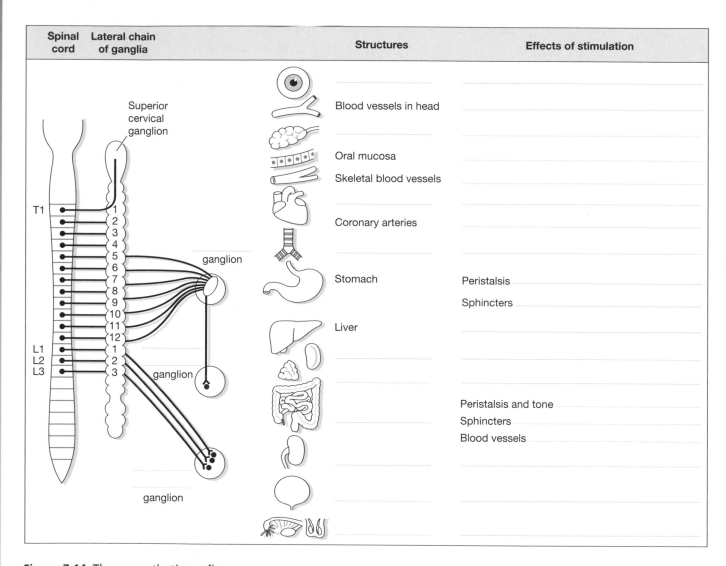

Figure 7.14 The sympathetic outflow

Colouring and labelling

71. Draw in lines representing the postganglionic fibres on Figure 7.15.

72. Explain why only some of the organs on Figure 7.15 appear to have postganglionic parasympathetic fibres.

_____

_____

_____

_____

73. Colour and label the structures innervated by the parasympathetic nervous system.

74. Complete Figure 7.15 by inserting the effects of parasympathetic stimulation in the right-hand column.

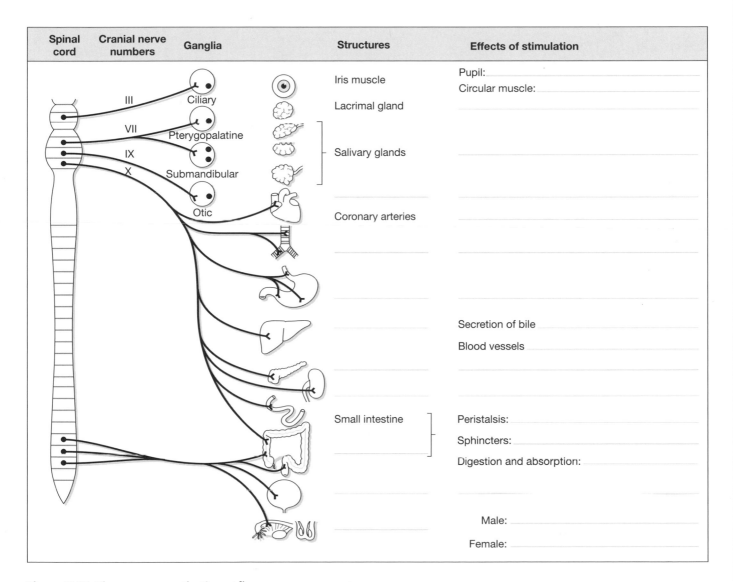

Figure 7.15 The parasympathetic outflow

Colouring and matching

15. Colour and match the photoreceptors on Figure 8.7:

○ Rod shaped nerve cell
○ Cone shaped nerve cell

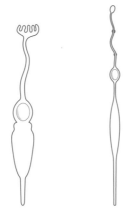

Figure 8.7 Rods and cones

 ## Completion

16. Fill in the blanks to describe the interior of the eye.

The anterior segment of the eye is incompletely

divided into the _____ and _____

chambers by the _____. Both chambers contain

_____ secreted into the _____

chamber by the _____. It circulates in

front of the _____ and through the _____

into the _____ chamber and returns to the

circulation through the _____. As

there is continuous production and drainage, the

intraocular pressure remains fairly constant. The

structures in the front of the eye including the

_____ and the _____ are supplied with

nutrients by the _____. The posterior

segment of the eye lies behind the _____ and

contains the _____. It has the consistency

of _____ and provides sufficient intraocular

pressure to keep the eyeball from collapsing.

 ## Labelling

17. Identify the parts of the optic pathways shown in Figure 8.8.

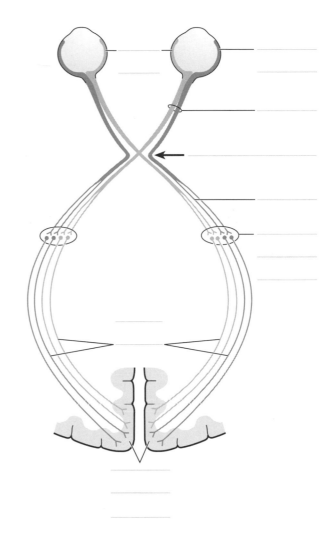

Figure 8.8 The optic nerves and their pathways

? MCQs

18. Light waves travel at the speed of: _____.

    a. 300 000 metres per second   **c.** 300 000 kilometres per second
    b. 300 000 metres per hour   **d.** 300 000 kilometres per hour.

19. Light waves of which colour have the shortest wavelength? _____.

    a. Red   **b.** Yellow   **c.** Violet   **d.** Blue.

20. When light waves pass from a medium of one density to another they bend. This process is called: _____.

    a. Reflection   **b.** Radiation   **c.** Refraction   **d.** Accommodation.

21. Which of the following structures causes the most significant bending of light waves? _____.

    a. Conjunctiva   **b.** Cornea   **c.** Lens   **d.** Vitreous body.

Matching and labelling

22. Insert the key choices into the appropriate spaces on the electromagnetic spectrum shown in Figure 8.9.

> *Key choices:*
> UV (ultraviolet) waves   Microwaves
> Radio waves   Gamma rays
> X-rays   Infrared rays

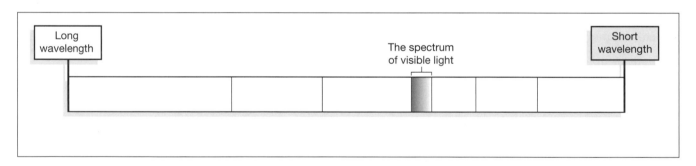

Figure 8.9 The electromagnetic spectrum

Colouring and matching

23. Colour and match the following parts of Figure 8.10A:

○ Ciliary body
○ Lens
○ Vitreous body

24. Label the two structures indicated on Figure 8.10A.

25. Complete Figure 8.10B by drawing in the changes that take place for near vision.

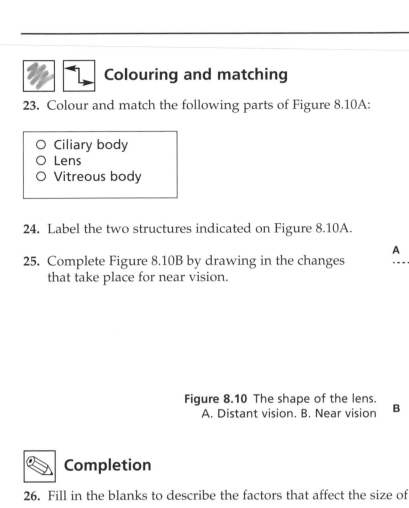

A

Figure 8.10 The shape of the lens. A. Distant vision. B. Near vision   **B**

Completion

26. Fill in the blanks to describe the factors that affect the size of the pupils.

The amount of light entering the eye is controlled by the _____ of the pupils. In a bright light they are

_____ and in darkness they are _____. The iris consists of two layers of smooth muscle –

contraction of the circular fibres causes _____ of the pupil while contraction of the radiating fibres causes

_____. The autonomic nervous system controls the size of the pupil – sympathetic stimulation causes

_____ while parasympathetic stimulation causes _____ of the pupil.

Pot luck

27. Name the three adjustments that the eyes make to focus on near objects (accommodation):

- _____
- _____
- _____.

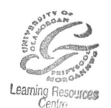

Completion

28. Complete Table 8.1 by inserting the action of each of the extrinsic muscles of the eye.

Extrinsic muscle	Action
Medial rectus	
Lateral rectus	
Superior rectus	
Inferior rectus	
Superior oblique	
Inferior oblique	

Table 8.1 Actions of the extrinsic muscles of the eye

   Colouring, matching and labelling

29. Colour, match and label the following on Figure 8.11:

- ○ Lacrimal gland
- ○ Upper and lower eyelids
- ○ Maxilla
- ○ Frontal bone
- ○ Optic nerve
- ○ Vitreous body
- ○ Lens
- ○ Tarsal plates

30. Emphasize the conjunctiva brightly.

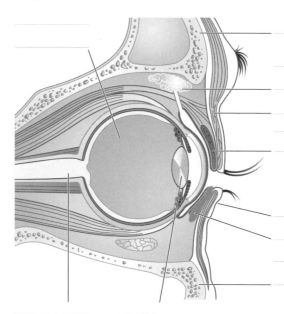

Figure 8.11 Section of the eye and its accessory structures

 Pot luck

31. List the constituents of tears: _____

_____.

32. State four functions of tears:

- ● _____
- ● _____
- ● _____
- ● _____.

SENSE OF SMELL

Pot luck

33. There are *five* errors in the paragraph below. Identify and correct them.

All odorous materials give off inert molecules that are carried into the nose in the inhaled air and stimulate the olfactory osmoreceptors. When currents of air are carried to the olfactory tract the smell receptors are stimulated, setting up impulses in the olfactory nerve endings. These pass through the cribriform plate of the mandible to the olfactory bulb. Nerve fibres that leave the olfactory bulb form the olfactory tract. This passes posteriorly to the olfactory lobe of the cerebellum where the impulses are interpreted and odour perceived.

Definitions

Define the following:

34. Anosmia _____

_____ .

35. 'Adaption' to smell _____

_____

_____ .

SENSE OF TASTE

Completion

36. Fill in the blanks in the paragraph below describing the sense of taste.

Taste buds contain sensory receptors called _____. They are situated in the papillae of the _____ and in the epithelia of the tongue, _____, _____ and _____. Some of the taste buds have hair-like _____ on their free border projecting towards tiny pores in the epithelium. Sensory receptors are stimulated by chemicals dissolved in _____ and _____ are generated when stimulation occurs. These are conducted to the brain where taste is perceived by the _____ area in the _____ lobe of the cerebral cortex.

Colouring and matching

37. Colour and match the following parts of taste buds on Figure 8.12B:

○ Taste cells

○ Supporting cells

○ Nerve fibres

○ Epithelial cells of the tongue

38. Draw in the taste 'hairs'.

39. List four different tastes that we perceive:

- _____
- _____
- _____
- _____.

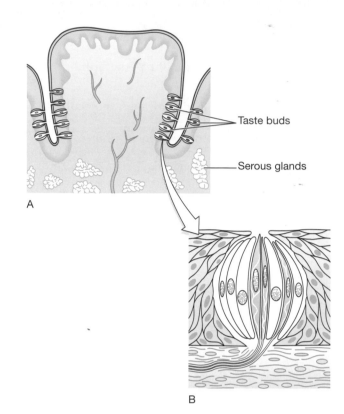

Taste buds

Serous glands

A

B

Figure 8.12 Structure of taste buds. A. A section of a papilla. B. A taste bud – greatly magnified

 ## Definitions

Define the following terms:

40. Astigmatism

_____
_____
_____
_____.

41. Myopia

_____
_____
_____
_____.

42. Hypermetropia

_____
_____
_____
_____.

 ## Applying what you know

43. Draw in the lenses and altered light waves that will correct the refractive errors of the eye to complete Figures 8.13C and E.

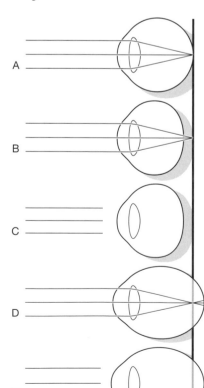

A

B

C

D

E

Figure 8.13 Common refractive errors of the eye and corrective lenses. A Normal eye. B and C Farsightedness. D and E Nearsightedness

9 The endocrine system

The endocrine system consists of ductless glands that secrete hormones. Together with the autonomic nervous system, the endocrine system maintains homeostasis of the internal environment and controls involuntary body functions. This chapter will help you explore the components of the endocrine system and their functions.

  Colouring and matching

1. Colour and match the endocrine glands identified on Figure 9.1:

○ Adrenal glands   ○ Pituitary gland
○ Ovaries (in female)   ○ Testes (in male)
○ Pancreatic islets   ○ Thymus gland
○ Pineal body   ○ Thyroid gland
○ Parathyroid glands

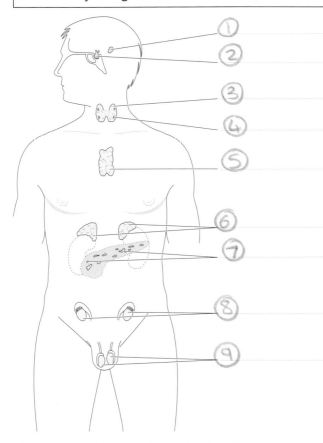

Figure 9.1 Positions of the endocrine glands

2. How many parathyroid glands are there?_____.
3. Describe the location of the parathyroid glands:

_____

_____.

Matching

4. Match the key choices to the spaces in the paragraph below to provide an overview of hormones.

Key choices:
Fast   Slow
Peptides   Receptor
Target organ   Polypeptides
Internal   Bloodstream
Secretes   Steroids
Proteins

A hormone is formed in one organ that _____

it into the _____ which then transports it to

its _____. When a hormone arrives at its

site of action, it binds to specific molecular groups on

the cell membrane called the _____. Homeostasis

of the _____ environment is maintained partly

by the _____ nervous system and partly

by the endocrine system. The former is concerned with

_____ changes while those that involve the

endocrine system are _____ and more precise

adjustments. Chemically, hormones fall into two

groups: _____ and _____.

Hormones in the first group are _____ soluble and

include _____ and _____. The latter

group includes _____ and _____.

PITUITARY GLAND AND HYPOTHALAMUS

 Matching

5.   Match the key choices to the statements in Table 9.1.

Key choices:

Anterior lobe of the pituitary	Pituicyte
Posterior lobe of the pituitary	Pituitary stalk
Intermediate lobe of the pituitary	Hypophyseal fossa
Adenohypophysis	Hypothalamus
Neurohypophysis	Pituitary portal system

Posterior lobe of the pituitary gland	
Anterior lobe of the pituitary gland	
Connects the pituitary gland to the hypothalamus	
Composed of glandular tissue	
Composed of nervous tissue	
Part of the pituitary whose function is unknown in humans	
Transports blood from the hypothalamus to the anterior pituitary	
Situated superiorly to the pituitary gland	
A hollow in the sphenoid bone	
A supporting cell of the posterior pituitary	

Table 9.1 Anatomy of the pituitary gland

Completion

6. Complete Table 9.2 by adding the full names and functions of anterior pituitary hormones.

Hormone	Abbreviation	Function
	GH	
	TSH	
	ACTH	
	PRL	
	FSH	Males: Females:
	LH	Males: Females:

Table 9.2 Summary of the hormones secreted by the anterior pituitary gland

 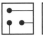 ## Labelling and completion

7. Name the structures identified in Figure 9.2.

8. Identify the eight hormones secreted by the pituitary gland in the box under Figure 9.2.

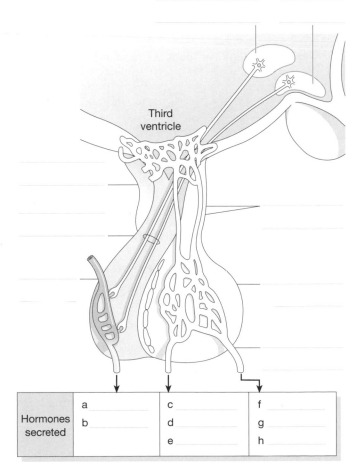

Third ventricle

Hormones secreted	a _____ b _____	c _____ d _____ e _____	f _____ g _____ h _____

Figure 9.2 The pituitary gland

Completion

9. Complete the boxes labelled a and b in Figure 9.3.

10. Match the hormones and effects from the key choices with the numbered parts of Figure 9.3.

Key choices:
Trophic hormones
Releasing hormones
Lowered
Raised

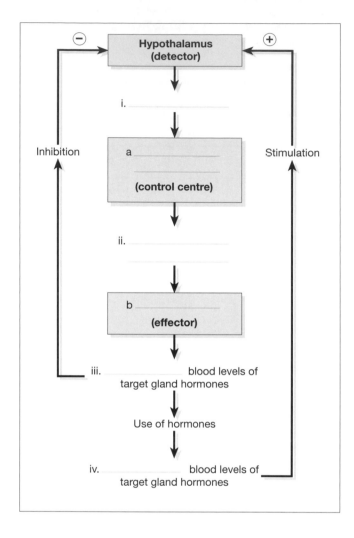

Figure 9.3 Negative feedback regulation of secretion of hormones

 MCQs

11. Release of which hormones varies during a 24-hour period (choose all that apply)? _____.

   a. Growth hormone   **b.** Thyroid stimulating hormone   **c.** Adrenocorticotrophic hormone   **d.** Prolactin.

12. Levels of which hormones are controlled by negative feedback mechanisms (choose all that apply)? _____.

   a. Growth hormone   **b.** Thyroid stimulating hormone   **c.** Adrenocorticotrophic hormone   **d.** Prolactin.

13. Levels of which hormone are controlled by a positive feedback mechanism? _____.

   a. Growth hormone   **b.** Thyroid stimulating hormone   **c.** Adrenocorticotrophic hormone   **d.** Prolactin.

14. Which is the most abundant hormone secreted by the anterior pituitary? _____.

   a. Growth hormone   **b.** Thyroid stimulating hormone   **c.** Adrenocorticotrophic hormone   **d.** Prolactin.

15. Secretion of which hormone peaks in adolescence? _____.

   a. Growth hormone   **b.** Thyroid stimulating hormone   **c.** Adrenocorticotrophic hormone   **d.** Prolactin.

16. Circadian rhythm means that regular fluctuations in hormone levels occur over a period of: _____.

    a. one hour   **b.** 24 hours   **c.** one week   **d.** one month.

17. Growth hormone stimulates (choose all that apply): _____.

    a. Absorption of calcium   **b.** Storage of fats   **c.** Division of body cells   **d.** Protein synthesis.

18. T_3 is also known as: _____.

    a. Thyroglobulin   **b.** Thyroxine   **c.** Tri-iodothyronine   **d.** Thyroid stimulating hormone.

Matching

19. Complete the paragraph below using the key choices listed, to provide an account of the effects of oxytocin:

Key choices:
Key choices:
Myoepithelial cells
Stimulation
Hypothalamus
Lactation
Parturition
Positive
Posterior pituitary
Stimulates
Stretch receptors
Uterine cervix
Smooth muscle

Oxytocin stimulates two target tissues before and after childbirth. These are uterine _____ and

_____ of the lactating breast. During childbirth, also known as _____, increasing amounts

of oxytocin are released in response to increasing _____ of sensory _____ in the

_____ by the baby's head. Sensory impulses are generated and travel to the _____

stimulating the _____ to secrete more oxytocin. This _____ the uterus to contract more

forcefully moving the baby's head further downwards through the uterine cervix and vagina. The mechanism

stops shortly after the baby has been born. This is an example of a _____ feedback mechanism. After birth

oxytocin stimulates _____.

THYROID GLAND

 Matching

20. Match the key choices from the list with the statements in Table 9.3 to describe the structure of the thyroid gland.

Key choices:		
Iodine	The thyroid gland is surrounded by this structure	
Isthmus	Joins the two thyroid lobes together	
Parathyroid glands	Lie against the posterior surface of the thyroid gland	
Parafollicular cells	Secrete the hormone calcitonin	
Thyroglobulin	Constituent of T_3 and T_4	
TSH	Secreted by the hypothalamus	
TRH	Thyroxine	
T_4	Precursor of T_3 and T_4	
Recurrent larnygeal	Secreted by the anterior pituitary	
Capsule	The nerves close to the thyroid gland	

Table 9.3 Features of the thyroid gland

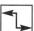 **Colouring and matching**

21. Colour and match the parts of the thyroid gland shown in Figure 9.4:

○ Blood vessels
○ Follicles
○ Follicular cells
○ Interlobular connective tissue
○ Parafollicular cells

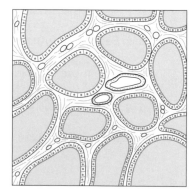

Figure 9.4 The microscopic structure of the thyroid gland

Completion

22. Complete Table 9.4 to summarize the effects of excess and deficiency of T_3 and T_4.

Body function affected	Hypersecretion of T_3 and T_4	Hyposecretion of T_3 and T_4
Metabolic rate		
Weight		
Appetite		
Mental state		
Scalp		
Heart		
Skin		
Faeces		
Eyes		None

Table 9.4 Effects of abnormal secretion of thyroid hormones

PARATHYROID GLANDS

 Colouring and matching

23. Colour and match the structures indicated on Figure 9.5:

- ○ Arteries
- ○ Veins
- ○ Oesophagus
- ○ Parathyroid glands
- ○ Thyroid gland
- ○ Pharynx
- ○ Recurrent pharyngeal nerves

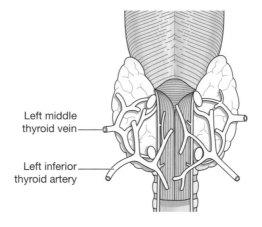

Left middle thyroid vein

Left inferior thyroid artery

Figure 9.5 The positions of the parathyroid glands and their related structures, viewed from behind

Pot luck

24. Identify the five mistakes in the paragraph below and correct them.

The parathyroid glands secrete parathyroid hormone (PTH, prothyroid hormone). Blood calcium levels regulate its secretion. When they rise, secretion of PTH is increased and vice versa. The main function of PTH is to decrease the blood calcium level. This is achieved by decreasing the amount of calcium absorbed from the small intestine and reabsorbed from the renal tubules. Normal blood calcium levels are needed for muscle relaxation, blood clotting and nerve impulse transmission.

ADRENAL GLANDS

 Matching

25. Match the key choices below with the statements in Table 9.5 to complete characteristics of the adrenal glands.

Key choices:	
Aldosterone	Kidneys
Androgens	Suprarenal
Medulla	Hydrocortisone
Cortex	Cholesterol

Is essential for life	
Inner part of the adrenal gland	
Veins that drain the adrenal glands	
The organs immediately inferior to the adrenal glands	
Male sex hormones	
The lipid that forms the basic structure of adrenocorticoids	
A mineralocorticoid hormone	
A glucocorticoid hormone	

Table 9.5 Features of the adrenal glands

Completion

26. Identify the structures labelled a, b, c and d on Figure 9.6.

27. Insert an arrow in each circle on Figure 9.6 to indicate whether the response to stress is to increase or decrease each effect.

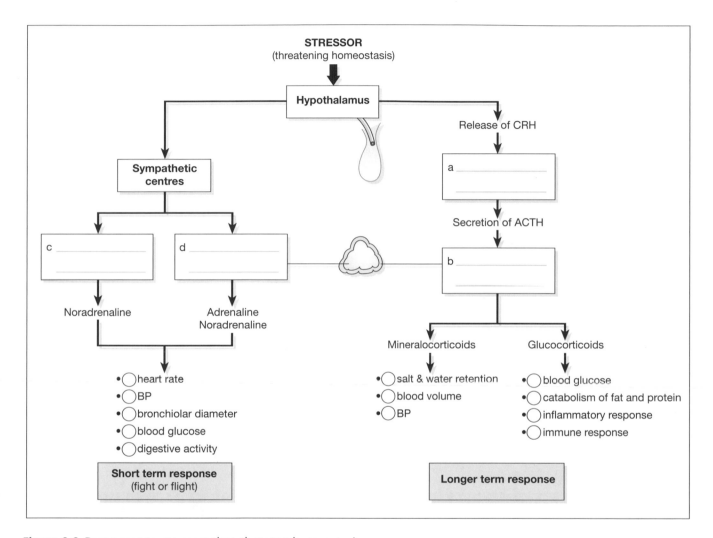

Figure 9.6 Responses to stressors that threaten homeostasis

PANCREATIC ISLETS

 Pot luck

28. Name the pancreatic cells that secrete these hormones:

   a. Insulin: _____

   b. Glucagon: _____

   c. Somatostatin: _____ .

29. State whether each statement below is TRUE or FALSE:

a. Insulin is formed from amino acids: _____

b. Normal blood glucose levels range from 6.1 to 9.9 mmol/litre: _____

c. nsulin reduces blood glucose levels: _____

d. Glucagon reduces blood sugar levels: _____

e. Secretion of insulin is stimulated by low blood sugar levels: _____

f. Secretion of insulin is stimulated by gastrin: _____

g. The hypothalamus is involved in secretion of insulin: _____

h. Insulin secretion is decreased by sympathetic stimulation: _____.

Completion

30. Enter the effect of each pathway on metabolism in the middle column of Table 9.6.

31. In the right-hand column enter the hormone that stimulates the pathway – insulin or glucagon.

Metabolic pathway	Effect of pathway on metabolism	Stimulated by insulin or glucagon?
Gluconeogenesis		
Lipogenesis		
Glycogenesis		
Glycogenolysis		
Lipolysis		

Table 9.6 The effect of insulin and glucagon on metabolic processes

LOCAL HORMONES

 MCQs

32. Histamine is (choose all that apply): _____.

a. A bronchoconstrictor
b. Released as part of the inflammatory process
c. An enzyme
d. Involved in blood clotting.

33. Serotonin is (choose all that apply): _____.

a. An enzyme   b. A hormone   c. Present in platelets   d. Present in erythrocytes.

34. Prostaglandins are: _____.

a. Cells in the prostate gland
b. Long acting substances
c. Involved in the cardiac cycle
d. Involved in blood clotting.

35. The inflammatory process involves (choose all that apply): _____.

a. Histamine   b. Serotonin   c. Prostaglandins   d. Erythropoietin.

10 The respiratory system

The respiratory system is a collection of tissues and organs whose collective function is primarily oxygen intake and carbon dioxide elimination. Conventionally, the respiratory system is divided into the upper respiratory tract (those structures not contained within the chest) and the lower respiratory tract (those structures found inside the chest).

  Labelling and matching

1. Label the following parts of the respiratory system on Figure 10.1, using the following terms:

Nasal cavity	Base of left lung	Right secondary bronchus
Pharynx	Parietal pleura	Right primary bronchus
Epiglottis	Visceral pleura	Ribs
Larynx	Trachea	
Apex of right lung	Left primary bronchus	

  Colour and match

2. Colour and match the:

- ○ Diaphragm
- ○ Pleural cavity
- ○ Clavicles

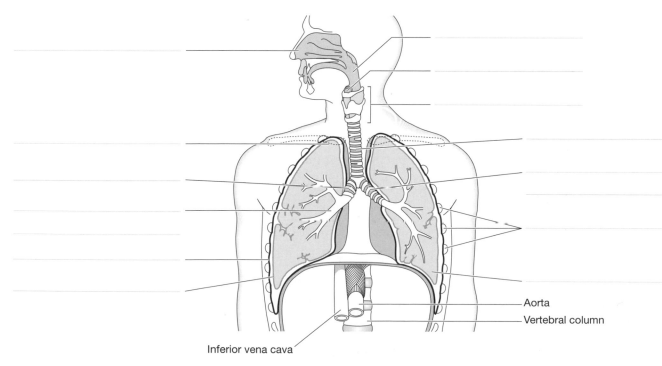

Figure 10.1 The organs of respiration

THE UPPER RESPIRATORY TRACT

 ### Matching

3. Match the structures below with their functions.

Functions		Structures
a. Increases surface area to moisten and warm air	....	Nasopharyngeal tonsil
b. Contains the vocal cords	....	Epiglottis
c. Forms the Adam's apple	....	Nasal conchae
d. The lid of the larynx, protecting the tracheal opening	....	Thyroid cartilage
e. Muscle flap in the roof of the mouth	....	Larynx
f. A collection of lymphoid tissue, involved in immunity	....	Auditory tube
g. Links the nasopharynx and middle ear	....	Soft palate

 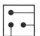 ### Colouring and labelling

4. Colour and label the structures in Figure 10.2.

- O Cricoid cartilage
- O Epiglottis
- O Thyroid cartilage
- O Hyoid bone
- O Thyrohyoid membrane
- O Rings of tracheal cartilage

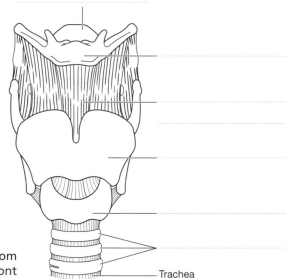

Figure 10.2 Larynx viewed from the front

Trachea

 ### Completion

5. Complete the following paragraph by inserting the correct word(s) in the spaces provided.

The upper respiratory passages carry air in and out of the respiratory system, but they have other functions too. The cells of their mucous membrane have _____, tiny hair-like structures that _____ in a wave-like motion towards the _____. They carry _____, which has been made by the _____ cells in the epithelial layer, and which traps _____ and _____ on its sticky surface. The air is therefore _____ by these mechanisms before it gets into the lungs. As the air passes through the nasal cavity, it is also _____ and _____ as it passes over the nasal _____, bony projections covered in mucous membrane. The nasal cavity also contains _____, which is covered in _____, and acts as a coarse filter for the air passing through. Immune tissue is present in patches called _____, which make _____ and therefore protect against inhaled antigens. Not only air passes through the pharynx, but also_____ and _____, and the tracheal opening is barricaded against these by the _____ .

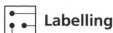 **Labelling**

6. Label the structures shown on Figure 10.3.

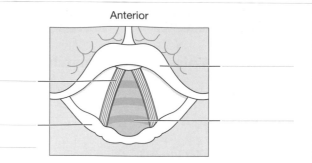
Anterior

Figure 10.3 Interior of the larynx viewed from above

? **MCQs**

7. One of the following options describing the vocal cords is true – which one? _____.

   a. The vocal cords are bands of membrane guarding the entrance to the oesophagus
   b. When the muscles controlling the vocal cords contract, the gap between the cords widens
   c. Speech is produced when air passing into the lungs vibrates the vocal cords
   d. When not in use, the vocal cords lie close together, i.e. are adducted.

8. Which of the following is not a function of the larynx? _____.

   a. A common passageway for food, air and water
   b. Modulation of speech
   c. Closing off of the lower respiratory tract by the epiglottis
   d. Humidification of air being breathed into the lungs.

9. The thyrohyoid membrane: _____.

   a. Lies anteriorly to the epiglottis   **c.** Vibrates to generate speech
   b. Links the hyoid bone to the thyroid gland   **d.** Forms part of the floor of the larynx.

10. Which of the following statements is true? _____.

    a. The larynx is built mainly of smooth muscle
    b. The epiglottis must be closed when speaking
    c. The larynx lies below the oropharynx
    d. The largest pieces of cartilage in the larynx are the arytenoids.

11. Which endocrine gland is closely associated with the larynx? _____.

    a. The pancreas   **b.** The thymus gland   **c.** The pineal gland   **d.** The thyroid gland.

THE LOWER RESPIRATORY TRACT

  Colouring and matching

12. On Figure 10.4, colour and match the following structures:

- ○ Oesophagus
- ○ Trachea
- ○ Tracheal cartilage rings

13. What shape are the tracheal cartilage rings?

_____

14. Why are they this shape?

_____

_____

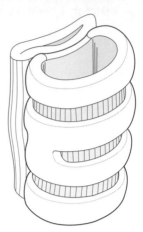

Figure 10.4 The relationship of the trachea to the oesophagus

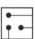 **Labelling**

15. Label the structures indicated on Figure 10.5.

16. There are two types of cell in this epithelial layer; identify them and state their functions:

Cell A: _____

_____.

Cell B: _____

_____.

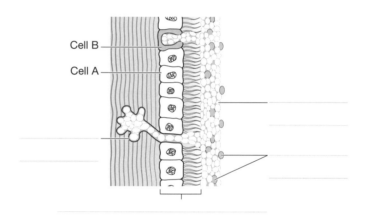

Figure 10.5 Microscopic view of ciliated mucous membrane

 Matching

17. For each of the four statements in list A, identify its most appropriate reason from list B. (You won't need all the items in list B.)

List A

Mucus is produced in the upper respiratory tract because...

_____

_____.

Cilia are present in the upper respiratory tract because...

_____

_____.

Cartilage is present in the upper respiratory tract because...

_____

_____.

Elastic tissue is present in the upper respiratory tract because...

_____

_____.

List B

... the passageway has to be flexible to allow head and neck movement

... the oesophagus is normally collapsed

... the oesophagus needs to expand during swallowing

... mucus needs to be swept away from the lungs

... the tissues need to return to their original shape

... this is an efficient way of removing dust and dirt from inhaled air

... mucus builds up during normal respiration

... the airways have to be kept open at all times

... inspired air must be warmed and humidified.

Pot luck

18. In the following paragraph, which describes the respiratory tree, there are *five* inaccuracies. Find them and correct them.

Ciliated respiratory epithelium lines the entire respiratory tree from the trachea to the alveoli, and its job is to keep the lungs clean. Cartilage rings support the airway walls; as the airways progressively divide and their diameter decreases, the amount of cartilage present increases. The smallest airways are called respiratory bronchioles, although no gas exchange takes place across their walls. The airways terminate in clusters of microscopic pouches called alveoli; it is here that most gas exchange takes place. The walls of the alveoli are necessarily very thin, and are only one cell thick; this layer contains macrophages, which make surfactant to keep the alveoli from collapsing. Gas exchange occurring across the alveolar walls is called internal respiration.

  Colouring, matching and labelling

19. In Figure 10.6, colour and label the structures indicated.

20. Colour and match the lobes of the lungs.

Right lung	*Left lung*
O Superior lobe	O Superior lobe
O Middle lobe	O Inferior lobe
O Inferior lobe	

21. Name the area between the lungs, in which the heart and other structures lie.

_____.

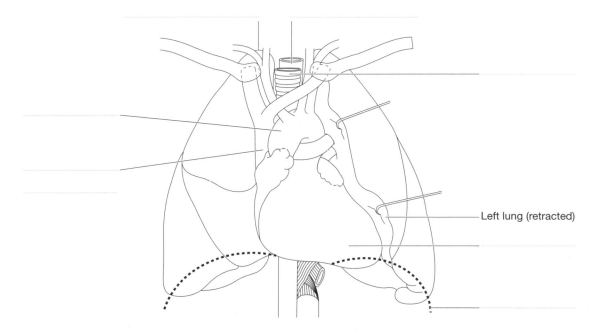

Left lung (retracted)

Figure 10.6 Organs associated with the lungs

Labelling

22. Label the visceral pleura, the parietal pleura, the pleural cavity, the diaphragm and the hilum of the right lung on Figure 10.7.

23. Where is the pleural fluid found, and what is its function? _____

_____

_____

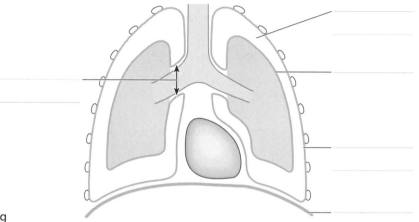

Figure 10.7 Relationship of pleura to the lung

? **MCQs**

24. The cough reflex is: _____.

    a. A voluntary protective response important in clearing airway obstruction
    b. Initiated by stimulation of sensory nerve endings in the upper airways
    c. Of no use in clearing normal airway mucus
    d. More efficient when the abdominal muscles are relaxed or weak.

25. Which of the following is true of autonomic innervation of the airways? _____.

    a. Sympathetic stimulation causes bronchoconstriction, and parasympathetic stimulation causes bronchodilation
    b. Sympathetic stimulation causes bronchodilation, and parasympathetic stimulation causes bronchoconstriction
    c. Both sympathetic and parasympathetic stimulation cause bronchoconstriction
    d. Both sympathetic and parasympathetic stimulation cause bronchodilation.

26. During the cough reflex: _____.
    a. Intra-abdominal pressure rises
    b. The glottis is collapsed
    c. The diaphram moves downwards
    d. There is, initially, a deep expiration.

27. Which of the following airways has the smallest diameter? _____.

    a. Respiratory bronchiole   **b.** Primary bronchus   **c.** Trachea   **d.** Tertiary bronchus.

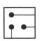 **Labelling and colouring**

28. As the respiratory tree progressively divides, the passageways become narrower and narrower. Label the structures on Figure 10.8. Indicate by colouring the large arrows the sections of the respiratory tree important in:

- ○ Air conduction
- ○ Gas exchange

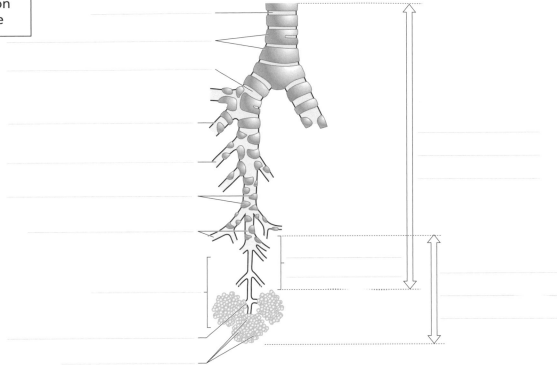

Figure 10.8 Lower respiratory tract

  Colouring and matching

29. On Figure 10.9, colour and match the:

- ○ alveolar endothelial cells
- ○ elastic connective tissue
- ○ blood capillaries.

30. Regarding Figure 10.9, complete the following sentences regarding cells A and B.

Cell A produces the substance that provides an oily lining for the alveolus; this substance

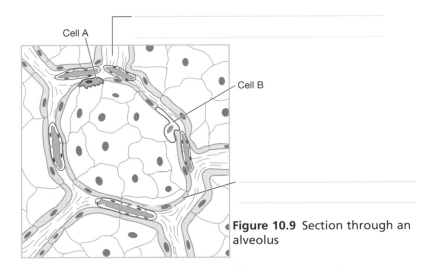

Figure 10.9 Section through an alveolus

is called _____ and the cell is a _____

_____ cell. Cell B is involved in protection; it cleans the alveolus by the process of

_____; it is a _____ .

Pot luck

31. Put the following statements in order, so that the flow of blood through the heart, lungs and systemic circulation is correctly summarized. The first one has been done to start you off.

Right ventricle	Body tissues
Pulmonary vein	Aorta
Pulmonary artery	Left ventricle
Lungs	Right atrium

1. Left atrium
↓
2. _____
↓
3. _____
↓
4. _____
↓
5. _____
↓
6. _____
↓
7. _____
↓
8. _____
↓
9. _____

RESPIRATION

 Completion

32. The paragraphs below describe a normal cycle of respiration. Fill in the blanks, using the terms supplied:

Passive	Increases	Inflate	Upwards
Deflate	Outwards	Muscular effort	Downwards
Inwards	Downwards	Into	Intercostal muscles
Relaxed	Decreases	Contracts	Increases
Relaxes	Intercostal muscles	Out of	Decreases

Just before inspiration commences, the diaphragm is _____; this occurs in the pause between breaths in normal quiet breathing. Inspiration commences. The ribcage moves _____ and _____ owing to contraction of the _____. The diaphragm _____ and moves _____. This _____ the volume of the thoracic cavity, and _____ the pressure. Because of these changes, air moves _____ the lungs, and the lungs _____. Inspiration has taken place.

    Unlike inspiration, expiration is usually a _____ process because it requires no _____. So, following the end of inspiration, the diaphragm _____ and moves back into its resting position. The ribcage moves _____ and _____, because the _____ have relaxed. This _____ the volume of the thoracic cavity, and so _____ the pressure within it. Air therefore now moves _____ the lungs, and they _____. There is now a rest period before the next cycle begins.

? MCQs

33. A lung that can be stretched easily but that does not return to its original shape is: _____.

    a. Elastic but not resistant
    b. Resistant but not compliant

    c. Compliant but not elastic
    d. Elastic but not compliant.

34. Compliance is: _____.

    a. The ability of the lung to stretch
    b. Very low in the normal healthy lung

    c. Another term for elasticity
    d. Increased when surfactant levels are low.

35. Elasticity is (choose all that apply): _____.

    a. The ability of the lung to stretch
    b. Very high in the normal healthy lung

    c. An opposing force to compliance
    d. Important in determining airways resistance.

36. Which of the following would decrease resistance in the healthy airway? _____.

    a. Increased goblet cell activity
    b. Parasympathetic activity

    c. Decreased pleural fluid production
    d. Relaxation of airway smooth muscle.

:: Labelling

37. Complete the list below, identifying each of the standard abbreviations for the main lung volumes and capacities, and use the abbreviations to label Figure 10.10:

    a. TV _____

    b. VC _____

    c. IC _____

    d. RV _____

    e. IRV _____

    f. ERV _____.

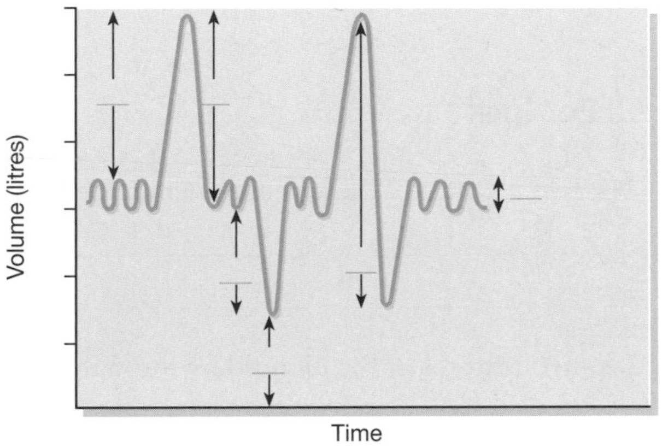

Figure 10.10 Lung volumes and capacities

✏ Applying what you know

38. If the functional residual capacity is 3000 ml, the tidal volume is 500 ml and the total lung capacity is 6000 ml, calculate the inspiratory capacity and the inspiratory reserve volume.

_____

39. If the total lung capacity is 6000 ml and the residual volume is 1200 ml, what is the vital capacity?

_____

40. Calculate the alveolar ventilation for an individual whose tidal volume is 450 ml, anatomical dead space is 160 ml and respiratory rate is 13/min.

_____

41. Emily is on the treadmill in the gym. Her pulse is 140/min, the tidal volume is 1200 ml, and her respiratory rate is 20/min. Of the volumes and capacities labelled in Figure 10.9, which two would be unchanged if you were to measure them right now? Explain your answers.

_____

_____

_____

_____

Definitions

Define the following terms:

42. External respiration: _____

_____

_____.

43. Internal respiration: _____

_____

_____.

Pot luck

44. List two features of the alveolar membrane that increase efficiency of gas exchange:

- _____
- _____.

45. List two features of the blood flow through the alveolar capillaries that increase efficiency of gas exchange:

- _____
- _____.

Colouring and completion

46. Fig. 10.11 shows gas exchange between an alveolus and a lung capillary.

    What is this process called?

    _____.

47. Using different colours for carbon dioxide and oxygen, colour in the arrows to show how each gas moves.

48. Complete the boxes to show the partial pressures of each gas in the arterial capillary, the venous capillary and the alveolus.

49. Colour the region on Fig. 10.11 that represents the respiratory membrane.

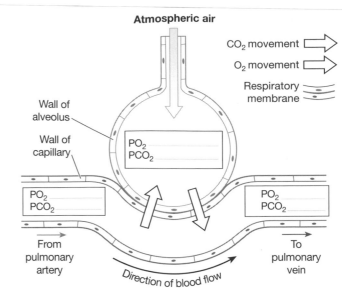

Figure 10.11 Gas exchange between alveoli and bloodstream

50. Fig. 10.12 shows gas exchange between the bloodstream and tissue cells.

    What is this process called? _____.

51. Using different colours for carbon dioxide and oxygen, colour in the arrows to show how each gas moves.

52. Complete the boxes to show the partial pressures of each gas in the arterial capillary, the venous capillary and the tissue cells.

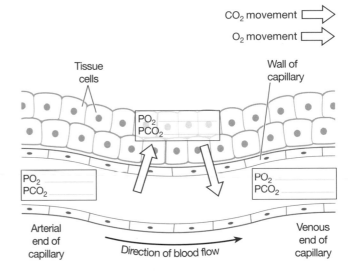

Figure 10.12 Gas exchange between the bloodstream and tissue cells

 MCQs

53. For normal gas exchange in the lung, which of the following is true? _____.

    a. Oxygen moves into the alveoli because the PO_2 is higher in the blood than in the alveoli
    b. Oxygen moves out of the alveoli because the PO_2 is higher in the alveoli than in the blood
    c. Oxygen moves into the alveoli because the PO_2 is higher in the alveoli than in the blood
    d. Oxygen moves out of the alveoli because the PO_2 is higher in the blood than in the alveoli.

54. For normal gas exchange in the lung, which of the following is true? _____.

    a. Carbon dioxide moves out of the alveoli because the PCO_2 is higher in the blood than in the alveoli
    b. Carbon dioxide moves out of the alveoli because the PCO_2 is higher in the alveoli than in the blood
    c. Carbon dioxide moves into the alveoli because the PCO_2 is higher in the alveoli than in the blood
    d. Carbon dioxide moves into the alveoli because the PCO_2 is higher in the blood than in the alveoli.

Matching

55. The following activity concerns internal respiration. Match the statements in list A with the best reason in list B. (You won't need all the reasons in list B, so choose carefully!)

List A

a. Carbon dioxide diffuses from the body cells into the bloodstream because …

_____.

b. Tissue levels of oxygen are lower than blood levels because …

_____.

c. Oxygen diffuses out of the capillary because …

_____.

d. The arterial end of the capillary is higher in oxygen than the venous end because …

_____.

List B

… blood flow is slow through the capillary beds

… PO_2 is lower in the tissues than in the bloodstream

… carbon dioxide is continually being produced by the tissues

… PCO_2 is lower in the capillary than in the tissues

… body cells require a constant supply of oxygen

… as the blood flows through the tissues it releases oxygen into the cells

… venous blood is deoxygenated

… body cells are continually using oxygen

TRANSPORT OF GASES

Pot luck

56. Decide whether the following statements apply to carbon dioxide, to oxygen, or to both.

   a. Waste product of metabolism: _____.

   b. 23% carried bound to haemoglobin: _____.

   c. Raised temperatures increase release from haemoglobin: _____.

   d. Mainly carried as bicarbonate ions in the plasma: _____.

   e. 98.5% carried bound to haemoglobin: _____.

   f. Binds loosely to haemoglobin: _____.

   g. Binding with haemoglobin is tighter in the lungs than in the tissues: _____.

   h. 1.5% carried dissolved in plasma: _____.

   i. Binding to haemoglobin is tighter in the tissues than in the lungs: _____.

CONTROL OF RESPIRATION

  Labelling and colouring

57. Label the structures indicated on Figure 10.13 using the items listed. Colour the nerve supply to the muscles of respiration.

Respiratory rhythmicity centre in medulla oblongata	Intercostal muscles
	Diaphragm
Cerebral cortex	Intercostal nerves
Glossopharyngeal nerve	Phrenic nerve
Spinal cord	Carotid body

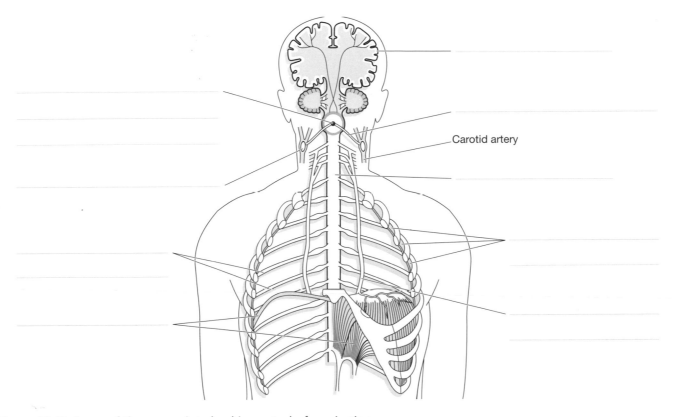

Carotid artery

Figure 10.13 Some of the nerves involved in control of respiration

Completion

58. Sort the list of stimuli in Table 10.1 according to whether they would increase or decrease respiratory effort. Place a tick in the appropriate column for each item.

Stimulus	Increases respiratory effort	Decreases respiratory effort
Fever		
Pain		
Sedative drugs		
Acidification of the CSF		
Sleep		
Exercise		
High blood [H⁺]		
Alkalinity of the blood		
Increased pH of the CSF		
Hypoxaemia		
Hypercapnia		
Stimulation of the respiratory centre		
Decreased CO_2 excretion		

Table 10.1 Causes of increased/decreased respiratory effort

? MCQs

59. Which one of the following is true of the chemical control of respiration? _____.

   a. Chemoreceptors are found only in the brain
   b. Chemoreceptors principally detect falling O_2 levels
   c. Central chemoreceptors are found in the cerebral cortex
   d. A fall in cerebrospinal fluid pH stimulates central chemoreceptors.

60. Which of the following are true (choose all that apply)? _____.

   a. The respiratory centre is located in the brainstem
   b. Accessory muscles of respiration include the diaphragm and the sternocleidomastoid
   c. Stimulation of the vagus nerve supplying aortic chemoreceptors increases the activity of the respiratory centre
   d. Control of breathing is entirely involuntary.

61. The Hering–Breuer reflex controls respiration by measuring: _____.

   a. Arterial blood pressure   c. CO_2 levels in the cerebrospinal fluid
   b. Airway resistance   d. Stretch in the lungs.

62. Which of the following is the key to why a child in a tantrum cannot hold his or her breath indefinitely? ____.

   a. Rising blood CO_2 levels   c. Rising blood pH
   b. Falling blood O_2 levels   d. Falling blood [H⁺].

11 Nutrition

All body cells need a supply of nutrients in appropriate quantities and the ultimate source of these nutrients is the diet. This chapter considers the main groups of nutrients and their roles in body function.

? Pot luck

1. List the six main nutrient groups needed for a balanced diet:

- _____
- _____
- _____
- _____
- _____
- _____.

Labelling and matching

2. Each section of the pyramid in Figure 11.1 represents a food group in their recommended proportions for a healthy diet. Label each of them, using the key choices below, and add three examples of each category.

Key choices:

A. Dairy products e.g.: _____
_____

B. Complex carbohydrates e.g.: _____
_____

C. Fruit and vegetables e.g.: _____
_____

D. Fats, oils and sweets e.g.: _____

E. Protein rich foods e.g.: _____
_____.

3. For each of the labelled sections, decide how many portions should be eaten daily in a balanced diet and write the answer in the appropriate part of the pyramid.

6–11 servings

5–9 servings

2–3 servings

2–3 servings.

Sparing

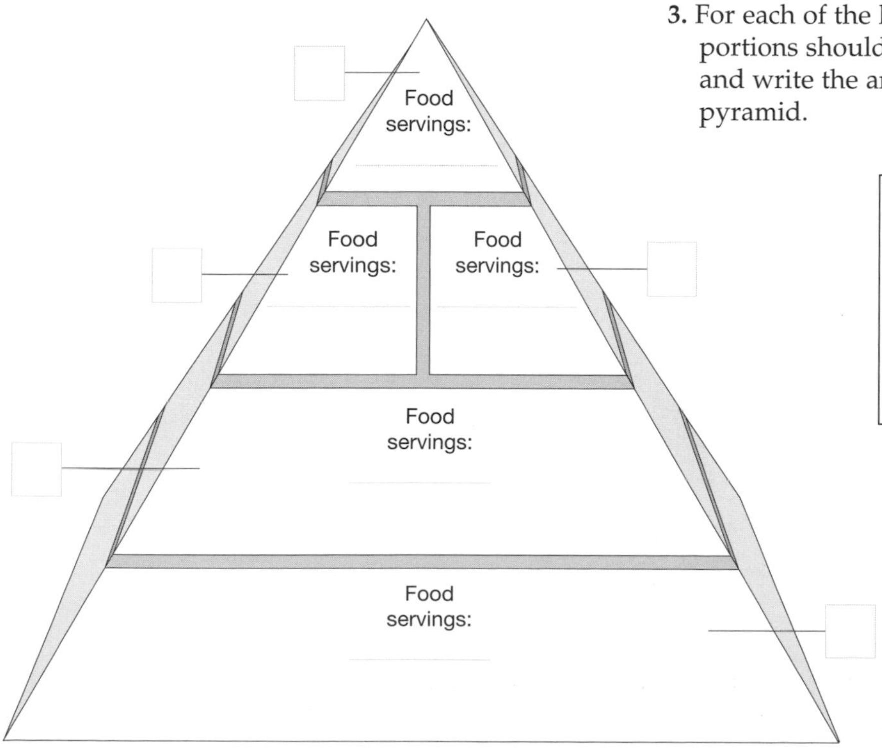

Food servings:

Food servings:

Food servings:

Food servings:

Food servings:

Figure 11.1 The main food groups and recommended proportions within a balanced diet

CARBOHYDRATES, PROTEINS AND FATS

? MCQs

4. Which of the following elements is/are found in carbohydrates (choose all that apply)? _____.

    a. Oxygen   **b.** Nitrogen   **c.** Hydrogen   **d.** Carbon.

5. A monosaccharide is (choose all that apply): _____.

    a. The simplest form in which sugars exist
    b. The form in which carbohydrate is absorbed from the small intestine
    c. A convenient form of carbohydrate storage
    d. The unit from which antibodies are made.

6. Cellulose is (choose all that apply): _____.

    a. The form in which carbohydrates are stored in the body   **c.** Found in fruit and vegetables
    b. A fat-based substance   **d.** Not digested in the human alimentary tract.

7. Which of the following is not true with regard to the use of carbohydrates in the body (choose all that apply)? _____.

    a. Carbohydrates are required for growth and repair of body tissues
    b. Carbohydrates are used as an energy source
    c. Excess dietary carbohydrate is stored as fat
    d. Carbohydrates can be converted to protein if the diet is low in protein.

📖 Definitions

Define the following terms:

8. Essential amino acid _____

_____.

9. Non-essential amino acid _____

_____.

10. Complete protein _____

_____.

? Pot luck

11. List the main functions of amino acids in the body:

    • _____

    • _____

    • _____.

✎ Completion

12. The following paragraph discusses the structure and function of the fats. Complete it by filling in the blanks.

The three elements that make up fat are _____, _____ and _____. Fats are usually divided into two groups: _____ fats are found in foods from animal sources, such as _____, _____ and _____. The second group, the _____ fats, are found in vegetable oils. Fat (adipose) tissue is laid down under the skin, where it acts as a(n) _____. It is also found around the kidneys, where its function is to _____ these organs. Fat depots in the body are important as _____ sources. Certain hormones, such as _____ e.g. cortisone, are synthesized from the fatty precursor _____, also found in the cell membrane. In addition, certain substances are absorbed with fat in the intestine, a significant example being the _____, which are essential for health despite being required only in very small amounts. Fats in a meal have the direct effect of _____ gastric emptying and _____ the return of a feeling of hunger.

THE VITAMINS AND MINERALS

13. Table 11.1 lists the main vitamins. Complete it by filling in the main dietary sources of each vitamin.

Vitamin	Main sources
A	
B_1 (thiamine)	
B_2 (riboflavine)	
Folate (folic acid)	
Niacin	
B_6 (pyridoxine)	
B_{12} (cyanocobalamin)	
Pantothenic acid	
Biotin	
C	
D	
E	
K	

Table 11.1 Vitamin sources

Matching

14. Vitamins act as cofactors in a range of important biochemical reactions in the body. Assign to each of the functions in list A the appropriate vitamin from list B. (You may need the items in list B more than once, and you can use more than one vitamin for each function.)

List A

a. Antioxidant: _____

b. Connective tissue synthesis: _____

c. Manufacture of visual pigments: _____

d. Non-essential amino acid synthesis: _____

e. Cell growth and differentiation, especially fast growing tissues: _____

f. Carbohydrate metabolism: _____

g. Synthesis of clotting factors: _____

h. DNA synthesis: _____

i. Amino acid/protein metabolism: _____

j. Regulation of calcium and phosphate levels: _____

k. Fat metabolism: _____

l. Myelin production: _____.

List B

Vitamin A

Vitamin B_1

Vitamin B_2

Vitamin B_6

Vitamin B_{12}

Folate (folic acid)

Pantothenic acid

Biotin

Niacin

Vitamin D

Vitamin E

Vitamin K

Vitamin C

15. The passage below describes the disorders that are associated with deficiency of certain vitamins. Complete it by deleting the incorrect options in bold, leaving the correct version.

Because vitamin A is a fat soluble vitamin, its absorption can be reduced if **bile/trypsin/pepsin** secretion into the gastrointestinal tract is lower than normal. The first sign of deficiency is **poor bone development/reduced immunity/night blindness**, and this may be followed by **poor blood clotting/conjunctival ulceration/neurological symptoms.** On the other hand, the B-complex vitamins are water soluble. Most of them are involved in **repair and differentiation of tissues/maintenance of an efficient immune system/biochemical release of energy.** Thiamine deficiency is associated with **pellagra/kwashiorkor/beriberi**, and niacin inadequacy leads to **pellagra/kwashiorkor/beriberi.** Folic acid is required for **DNA/collagen/clotting factor** synthesis, and is therefore often prescribed as a supplement in pregnancy. Deficiency of vitamin B_{12} typically leads to **haemolytic/megaloblastic/iron deficiency** anaemia, because it is needed for DNA synthesis, and is usually associated with lack of **biotin/bile/intrinsic factor** in the gastrointestinal tract.

Vitamin C is needed for **connective tissue synthesis/clotting factor synthesis/maintenance of normal bone tissue.** One of the first signs of deficiency of this vitamin is therefore loosening of the teeth, due to **defective gum tissue/bleeding into the gums because of clotting deficiency/erosion of the bony sockets.** Vitamin C is destroyed by **heat/water/low gastric pH.**

Lack of vitamin D causes **osteoporosis/osteoma/osteomalacia** in adults, and **scurvy/rickets/night blindness** in children. Vitamin E deficiency results in **haemolytic/megaloblastic/iron deficiency** anaemia, because the **cell membrane/haemoglobin content/cytoplasm** of red blood cells is damaged.

Vitamin K deficiency leads to problems with **myelination of nerves/absorption of calcium/blood coagulation.**

Matching

16. Complete Table 11.2 by ticking the appropriate boxes against each of the minerals shown.

	Calcium	Phosphate	Sodium	Potassium	Iron	Iodine
Needed for haemoglobin synthesis						
Used in thyroxine manufacture						
Most abundant cation outside cells						
99% of body stock is found in bones						
Most abundant cation inside cells						
May be added to table salt						
Vitamin D is needed for use						
Involved in muscle contraction						
Used to make high-energy ATP						
Needed for normal blood clotting						
Required for hardening of teeth						
Needed for normal nerve transmission						

Table 11.2 Functions of minerals

? **MCQs**

17. Where is dietary calcium mainly found (choose all that apply)? _____.

    a. Cheese   **b.** Milk   **c.** Drinking water   **d.** Meat products.

18. Where is dietary phosphate mainly found (choose all that apply)? _____.

    a. Cheese   **b.** Liver   **c.** Vegetables   **d.** Wholemeal bread.

19. Where is dietary sodium mainly found (choose all that apply)? _____.

    a. Processed foods   **b.** Oatmeal   **c.** Table salt   **d.** Meat.

20. Where is dietary potassium mainly found (choose all that apply)? _____.

    a. Fruit and vegetables   **b.** Table salt   **c .** Seafood   **d.** Meat.

21. Where is dietary iron mainly found (choose all that apply)? _____.

    a. Liver   **b.** Kidney   **c.** Red meat   **d.** Green vegetables.

22. Where is dietary iodine mainly found (choose all that apply)? _____.

    a. Vegetables   **b.** Meat products   **c.** Granulated sugar   **d.** Seafood.

FIBRE AND WATER

? Pot luck

23. NSP is the abbreviation for: _____

24. List the five main functions of NSP.

   • _____

   • _____

   • _____

   • _____

   • _____

25. What are the main dietary sources of NSP?

   • _____

26. What percentage of body weight is water in:

   • Men? _____

   • Women? _____.

12 The digestive system

The digestive system is a varied collection of organs and tissues, which participate in some way in the digestion and absorption of food. Food and drink taken orally is not usually in a chemically appropriate form for the tissues of the body to use, and the digestive system possesses a wide array of enzymes needed to convert what we eat and drink into a form more suitable for absorption and use.

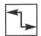   **Matching, colouring and labelling**

1. Figure 12.1 shows the digestive system.
   Match and colour the main parts using the key provided.

   ○ Rectum   ○ Duodenum
   ○ Liver   ○ Pancreas (behind stomach)
   ○ Stomach   ○ Oesophagus
   ○ Large intestine   ○ Gall bladder
   ○ Sigmoid colon   ○ Small intestine

2. Label the other structures indicated.

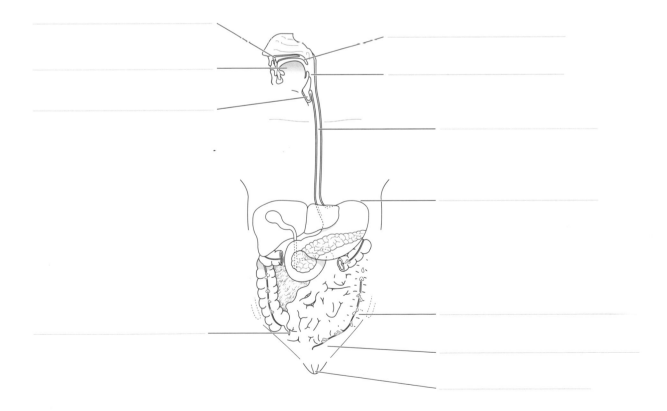

Figure 12. 1 The digestive system

Definition

Define the following term:

3. Enzyme _____

_____ .

? Pot luck

4. List the five processes that take place in the alimentary canal:

- _____
- _____
- _____
- _____
- _____ .

5. Distinguish between mechanical and chemical digestion:

_____

_____

THE BASIC STRUCTURE OF THE GASTROINTESTINAL TRACT

Matching

6. Decide whether the following structures are classed either as parts of the alimentary tract or accessory organs of digestion, and use them to complete Table 12.1.

Mouth	Liver	Gall bladder
Parotid glands	Stomach	Oesophagus
Pancreas	Submandibular glands	Sublingual glands
Small intestine	Large intestine	Rectum and anus

Organs of alimentary tract	Accessory organs

Table 12.1 Organs of the alimentary tract and accessory organs

Labelling, matching and colouring

7. Figure 12.2 shows a section through the wall of the alimentary canal, and although the digestive organs are varied in shape and function, this basic pattern is seen in almost all regions. Colour, match and label the nerve plexuses on Figure 12.2.

○ Myenteric (Auerbach's) plexus
○ Submucosal (Meissner's) plexus

8. Label the layers shown on Figure 12.2.

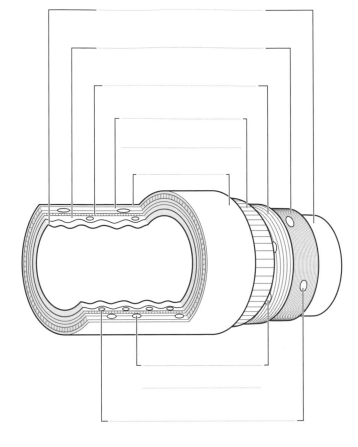

Figure 12.2 General structure of the alimentary canal

 MCQs

9. Which of the following statements concerning the peritoneum is true? _____.

   a. It contains many lymph nodes
   b. The visceral layer lines the abdominal cavity
   c. The uterus is covered only on its posterior surface
   d. The peritoneal cavity is lubricated with lymph.

10. What is the greater omentum? _____.

   a. The folds of peritoneum that anchor the liver to the diaphragm
   b. The visceral layer lines the abdominal cavity
   c. The extension of the peritoneum that hangs in front of the stomach
   d. The name given to the space between the two peritoneal layers.

11. Which of the following is not found in the mucosal layer of the alimentary canal? _____.

   a. Muscularis mucosa   b. Visceral peritoneum   c. Lamina propria   d. Mucus membrane.

12. Retroperiotoneal structures are situated: _____.

   a. Above the peritoneum
   b. Below the peritoneum
   c. Within the peritoneum
   d. Behind the peritoneum.

Labelling and colouring

13. What type of tissue is shown in Figure 12.3?

_____

14. Label the two cell types shown in the diagram, and colour and label the product of cell A.

15. Name two functions of the product of cell A:

- _____

- _____.

16. In which regions of the digestive tract is the tissue in Figure 12.3 found?

_____.

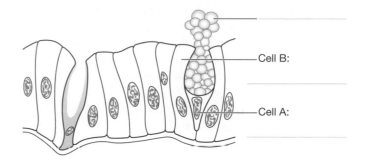

Figure 12.3 Cells of the digestive mucosa

THE UPPER GASTROINTESTINAL TRACT

 ## MCQs

17. Which of the following does not form part of the roof of the mouth? _____.

   a. The palatine bones   **c.** The maxillary bone
   b. The soft palate   **d.** The palatine tonsil.

18. The uvula is formed from: _____.

   a. Lymphoid tissue   **c.** Bone tissue
   b. Muscle tissue   **d.** Connective tissue.

19. Which of the following concerning the papillae is true? _____.

   a. The vallate papillae are the smallest of the taste buds
   b. Taste buds are found only at the front of the tongue
   c. Filiform papillae lie towards the back of the tongue
   d. Papillae at the tip of the tongue are mainly fungiform in type.

20. Which of the following statements concerning the tongue is true? _____.

   a. It is made of involuntary muscle   **c.** It is the only structure in the mouth possessing nerves for taste
   b. Its base is anchored to the hyoid bone   **d.** Its role in swallowing is minimal.

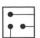 ## Labelling and colouring

21. Figure 12.4 shows the roof of the mouth complete with teeth. Label and colour the different teeth shown.

22. State the functions of the different types of teeth in Figure 12.4.

    A_____

    B_____

    C_____

    D_____

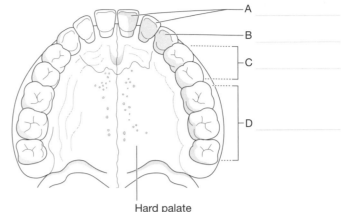

Hard palate

Figure 12.4 The roof of the mouth and the permanent teeth

  ## Labelling and colouring

23. Figure 12.5 shows the internal structure of a tooth. Label the structures indicated.

24. Colour the following parts on Figure 12.5 using the key, and describe the function and main characteristics of each.

    ○ Cement _____

    _____

    ○ Dentine _____

    _____

    ○ Enamel _____

    _____

25. What is found within the pulp cavity?

    _____

26. There are 32 permanent teeth and only 20 deciduous (baby) teeth. Name and number the teeth that are missing from a child's dentition.

    _____

    _____

    _____

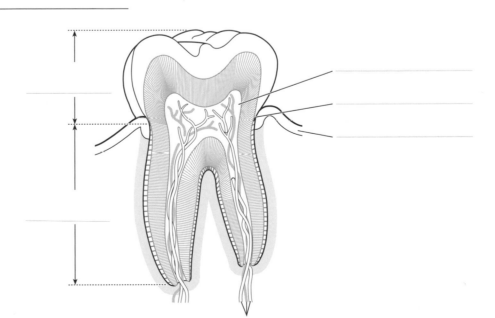

Figure 12.5 A section of a tooth

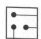   **Labelling, matching and colouring**

27. Figure 12.6 shows the position of the salivary glands. They are paired, so both sides of the mouth contain them. Label the structures indicated.

28. On Figure 12.6, colour and match the glands themselves using the key below and identify where the salivary glands open into the mouth.

○ _____ gland

opens into: _____

○ _____ gland

opens into: _____

○ _____ gland

opens into: _____

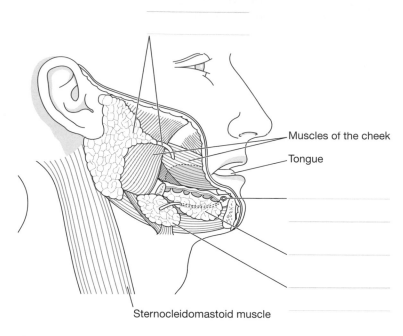

Muscles of the cheek

Tongue

Sternocleidomastoid muscle

Figure 12.6 Position of salivary glands

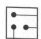 **Labelling**

29. Figure 12.7 shows the stomach and structures close by. Label the structures indicated.

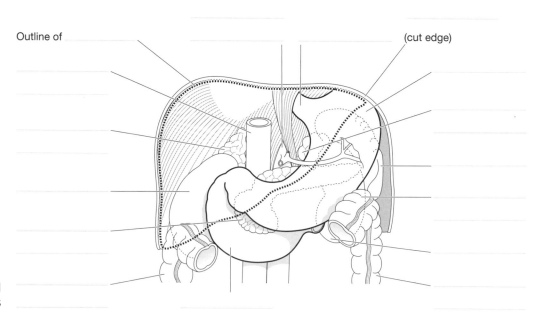

Outline of _____ (cut edge)

Figure 12.7 Stomach and associated structures

SMALL INTESTINE

Matching

39. The small intestine is divided into three sections: the duodenum, the jejunum and the ileum. For each of the statements in Table 12.2, decide to which section it applies by ticking the relevant box in the table.

	Duodenum	Jejunum	Ileum
Longest portion of the small intestine			
Curves around the head of the pancreas			
Vitamin B$_{12}$ is absorbed here			
About 25 cm long			
Middle section			
Ends at the ileocaecal valve			
Flow in is regulated by the pyloric sphincter			
Most digestion takes place here			
About 2 m long			
Flow from here enters the large intestine			
Bile passes into this section			
The pancreas passes its secretions into this section			
Villi present here			
Most absorption takes place here			

Table 12.2 Characteristics of the duodenum, jejunum and ileum

Labelling and colouring

40. Figure 12.9 shows a single villus, only one of the millions that line the small intestine, giving it a velvety appearance. Of the four layers of the wall of the tract, which one forms the villi?

_____

41. Label the main structures shown on Figure 12.9. Colour the arterial blood supply red, the venous drainage blue and the lymphatic vessels green.

42. What is absorbed into the central vessel of the villus?

_____

43. What is the name of the large collections of lymphoid tissue found in the intestine?

_____

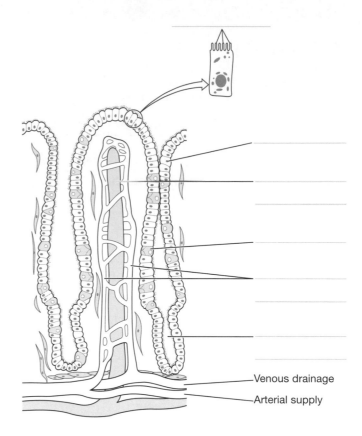

Venous drainage

Arterial supply

Figure 12.9 Highly magnified view of single villus

 Completion

44. The following passage describes chemical digestion in the small intestine. Complete it by scoring out the incorrect option(s) in bold, thus leaving the right one(s).

On a daily basis, the intestine secretes about **1500 ml/2000 ml/2500 ml** of intestinal juices, and its contents are **usually acidic, because the contents coming from the stomach are acidic/between 7.8 and 8.0/very alkaline, to neutralize stomach acid.** In the small intestine, chemical digestion is completed and the end products are absorbed. The main enzyme secreted by the enterocytes is enterokinase, which **breaks down proteins to polypeptides/activates enzymes from the pancreas/neutralizes stomach acid and stops the action of pepsin.** However, other enzymes from accessory structures are passed into the **duodenum/jejunum/ileum** as well.

The pancreas secretes **sucrase/amylase/maltase**, which is important in reducing large sugar molecules to **amino acids/glucose/disaccharides.** In addition, pancreatic lipase breaks down fats into **fatty acids and glucose/amino acids and glycerol/fatty acids and glycerol**, which can be absorbed in the intestine. The third major nutrient group, the proteins, are broken down to **amino acids/dipeptides/polypeptides** by pancreatic **trypsin and chymotrypsin/pepsin and trypsin/chymotrypsin and pepsin.** Pancreatic juice is also rich in **chloride/hydrogen/bicarbonate** ions, important in neutralizing the acid chyme from the stomach.

Bile is made in the **gall bladder/liver/duodenum**, stored in the **gall bladder/liver/duodenum**, and enters the intestine via the **cardiac sphincter/hepatopancreatic sphincter/biliary sphincter.** It has a role to play in fat digestion by breaking fats into **fatty acids and glycerol/tiny droplets/soluble ions.** This increases the action of lipases on the fat.

Even after the multiple digestive actions of these enzymes, the digested proteins and carbohydrates are still not in a readily absorbable form, and digestion is completed by enzymes made by the **enterocytes/goblet cells/lacteals.** Thus, the final stage of protein digestion produces **glucose/amino acids/dipeptides** and the final stage of carbohydrate digestion produces **monosaccharides/glycogen/sucrose.**

MCQs

45. Why does the pancreas secrete its proteolytic enzymes in an inactive form? _____.

    a. To reduce waste
    b. To prevent the active enzyme from digesting the duodenum
    c. To increase the body's control of the digestive processes
    d. To prevent pancreatic damage.

46. Which of the following statements concerning control of pancreatic secretion is true? _____.

    a. It is regulated by secretin and gastrin, which are made in the duodenum
    b. Secretin and cholecystokinin stimulate pancreatic secretion
    c. The stretching of the duodenal walls when food enters stimulates secretin release
    d. Gastrin is released directly into the pancreas from the enteroendocrine cells that secrete it.

47. Which of the following vitamins would be absorbed in reduced amounts if bile were absent from the intestine (choose all that apply)? _____.

    a. A   **b.** B   **c.** C   **d.** D.

48. Which hormone is released when a high fat meal has been eaten, and stimulates contraction of the gall bladder? _____.

    a. Bile   **b.** Cholecystokinin   **c.** Secretin   **d.** Gastrin.

 Labelling and completion

49. Figure 12.10 shows two intestinal villi that will absorb an assortment of the main nutrients.

    a. Label the parts shown.

    b. The three main nutrients – glucose, amino acids and fatty acids – are represented by different symbols in the key and on the figure. Complete the key, using the distribution of the symbols as a guide.

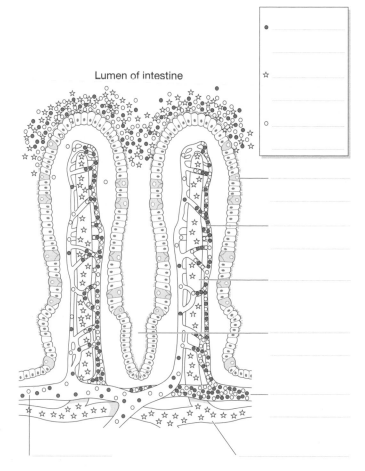

Figure 12.10 The absorption of nutrients

Pot luck

50. Into which vessel in the villus are the following vitamins absorbed?

A _____

B _____

C _____

D _____

E _____

K _____.

51. Some absorbed nutrients pass into the villus simply because there is more of them in the intestine than in the blood – this is simple diffusion. What is the other mechanism by which nutrients can be absorbed?

_____

52. Name three examples of molecules transported by the mechanism you have identified in question 51.

- _____
- _____
- _____.

 Completion

53. A huge volume of fluid is secreted into the gastrointestinal tract daily. Given an average daily fluid intake of 1200 ml, complete Figure 12.11, which summarises the average volumes of fluid secreted, absorbed and eliminated in 24 hours.

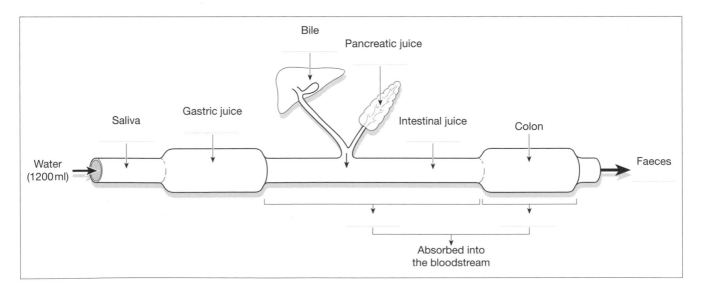

Figure 12.11 Average daily volumes of fluid in the gastrointestinal tract

LARGE INTESTINE, RECTUM AND ANAL CANAL

 MCQs

54. What are the taenia coli? _____.

    a. The anal sphincters that control the opening of the anus
    b. Bands of longitudinal muscle that pucker the colon
    c. Dense collections of submucosal lymphoid tissue
    d. The dense population of mucus secreting cells in the rectum.

55. What is the main substance absorbed in the colon? _____.

    a. Water   **b.** Sugars   **c.** Proteins   **d.** Fatty acids.

56. Which of the following statements concerning defaecation is true? _____.

    a. The anal columns allow contraction of the anal canal
    b. The anal sphincters are a continuation of the longitudinal muscle of the colon
    c. The internal anal sphincter is under conscious voluntary control
    d. The desire to defaecate is initiated by stimulation of stretch receptors in the rectum.

57. Which of the following statements concerning faeces is true? _____.

    a. The main constituent is fibrous and indigestible material
    b. The bacteria present are dead
    c. They are deodorized by stercobilin
    d. Their brown colour comes from the fatty content.

PANCREAS

Labelling and colouring

58. The pancreas and its associated structures are shown in Figure 12.12. Label and colour the structures indicated.

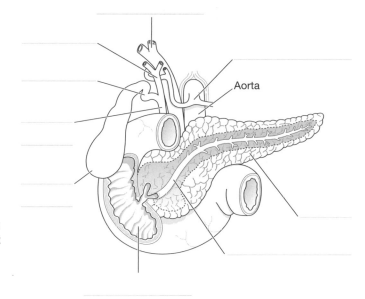

Figure 12.12 The pancreas in relation to the duodenum and biliary tract

Matching

59. The pancreas secretes two types of substances, and is considered both an exocrine and an endocrine gland. Complete Table 12.3 using the choices listed and summarize the functions of the pancreas.

Secretions leave via the pancreatic duct
Control of blood sugar levels
Substances are passed directly into blood
Role is in digestion
Synthesis takes place in pancreatic alveoli
Secretion of enzymes

Synthesis takes place in the pancreatic islets
Secretion of glucagon
Secretions include amylase, lipase and proteases
Secretion of hormones
Passes secretions into duodenum
Secretion of insulin

Exocrine functions	Endocrine functions

Table 12.3 Functions of the pancreas

THE LIVER AND THE BILIARY TRACT

  Colouring and matching

60. Figure 12.13 shows the anterior surface of the liver. Colour and match the following structures:

- ○ Right lobe
- ○ Left lobe
- ○ Gall bladder
- ○ Falciform ligament
- ○ Inferior vena cava

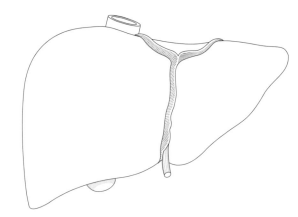

61. What structure lies immediately above the liver?

_____

Figure 12.13 Anterior view of liver

Labelling

62. Figure 12.14 shows a magnified transverse section of a liver lobule. Label the structures indicated.

63. In Figure 12.14, blood flows from the small peripheral vessels (shown in groups at the corners of the lobule and associated with a bile duct) towards the central vein in the middle of the lobule. There are two vessels, an artery and a vein. What is the significance of the fact that there is both an arterial and a venous supply to the liver?

_____

_____

_____

_____

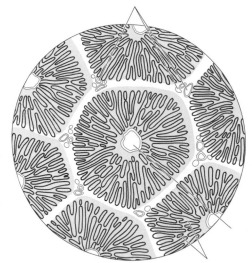

Figure 12.14 A magnified transverse section of a liver lobule

Completion

64. The following paragraphs describe the functions of the liver. Fill in the blanks.

The liver is involved in the metabolism of carbohydrates; it converts glucose to _____ for storage; the hormone that is important for this is _____. In the opposite reaction, glucose is released to meet the body's energy needs and the important hormone for this is _____. This action of the liver maintains the blood sugar levels within close limits. Other metabolic processes include the formation of waste, including _____, from the breakdown of protein, and _____ from the breakdown of nucleic acids. Transamination is the process by which _____ are made from _____. Proteins are also made here; two important groups of proteins, found in the blood, are the _____ and the _____.

The liver detoxifies many ingested chemicals, including _____ and _____. It also breaks down some of the body's own products, such as _____. Red blood cells and other cellular material such as microbes are broken down in the _____ cells. It synthesizes vitamin ____ from _____, a provitamin found in plants such as carrots, and stores it, along with other vitamins. The liver is also the main storage site of _____ (essential for haemoglobin synthesis).

The liver makes _____, which is stored in the gall bladder and important in digestion of _____. Bile salts are important for _____ in the small intestine, and are themselves reabsorbed there and returned to the liver in the _____. This is called the _____ circulation, and helps to conserve the body's store of bile salts. Bilirubin is released when _____ are broken down (this occurs mainly in the _____ and the _____). Bilirubin is not very soluble so, to increase its water solubility so that it can be excreted in the bile, it is conjugated with _____. On its passage through the intestine, it is converted by bacteria to _____, which is excreted in the faeces; some is, however, reabsorbed and excreted in the urine as _____. If levels of bilirubin in the blood are high, its yellow colour is seen in the tissues as _____.

Labelling, matching and colouring

65. Figure 12.15 shows the gall bladder, bile ducts and their connections with the duodenum. Label the structures indicated.

66. Insert arrows in one colour to show the direction of flow of bile from the liver into the gall bladder for storage, and in another colour to show the direction of flow from the gall bladder into the duodenum.

> ⇨ – Flow from liver to gall bladder
> ⇨ – Flow from gall bladder to duodenum

67. Colour and match the following.

> ○ Gall bladder
> ○ Duodenum
> ○ Pancreas

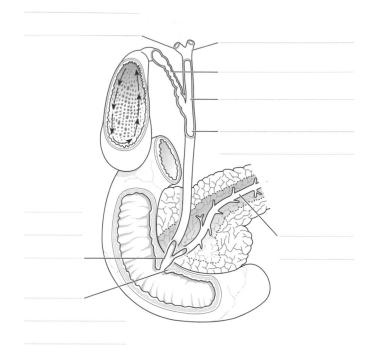

Figure 12.15 Flow of bile from liver to duodenum

? **MCQs**

68. Which section of the biliary tract does bile have to pass through twice? _____.

  a. Hepatic duct   **b.** Biliary duct   **c.** Cystic duct   **d.** Common bile duct.

69. Which of the following statements concerning the gall bladder is true? _____.

  a. Bile is concentrated because water is absorbed through the gall bladder wall
  b. The two layers of muscle in the wall of the gall bladder contract to expel bile
  c. Fatty and acid chyme in the stomach stimulates release of bile
  d. Sympathetic activity in the gall bladder nerve supply stimulates bile release.

70. Which of the following is not found in bile? _____.

  a. Water   **b.** Mucus   **c.** Lipase   **d.** Cholesterol.

71. The volume of bile secreted daily is: _____.

  a. 200 ml   **b.** 800 ml   **c.** 500 ml   **d.** 300 ml.

METABOLISM

📖 Definitions

Define the following terms:

72. Catabolism _____

_____.

73. Anabolism _____

_____.

74. Explain the difference between a kilocalorie and a kilojoule.

_____

_____

❓ MCQs

75. Which of the following concerning the basal metabolic rate (BMR) is true? _____.

    a. The individual should not have eaten within 6 hours of the test
    b. The BMR is independent of age or body weight
    c. The BMR reflects the level of energy production needed for only the most vital of body functions
    d. Reduction in food intake increases the BMR and causes loss of body weight.

76. The end result of energy producing metabolic pathways is the production of which high-energy molecule? ____.

    a. Glucose   **b.** Glycogen   **c.** Citric acid   **d.** Adenosine triphosphate.

77. Which is the preferred fuel molecule for cellular production of energy? _____.

    a. Glucose   **b.** Glycogen   **c.** Citric acid   **d.** Adenosine triphosphate.

78. Normal blood sugar levels are: _____.

    a. 2–5 mmol/l   **b.** 5–8 mmol/l   **c.** 8–11mmol/l   **d.** 11–14 mmol/l.

79. What happens to excess glucose in the body (choose all that apply)? _____.

    a. It is excreted in the urine   **c.** It is converted to glucagon
    b. It is converted to fat   **d.** It is stored in liver and skeletal muscle in a polymerized form.

80. Gluconeogenesis is an important metabolic process because it is the: _____.

    a. Use by body cells of non-carbohydrate sources of energy, e.g. fats or proteins
    b. Production of glycogen from glucose for energy storage
    c. Conversion of molecules other than carbohydrates to glucose
    d. Production of ATP from energy sources such as glucose and other carbohydrates.

Labelling, matching and colouring

81. Figure 12.16 shows the biochemical fate of glucose in the cell both in the presence and absence of oxygen. Colour, match and label the arrows to show the three main pathways.

○ Glycolysis
○ Citric acid (Krebs') cycle
○ Oxidative phosphorylation

82. Complete the pathways by inserting the correct metabolic intermediates and products in the spaces provided.

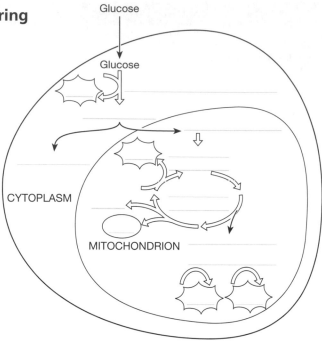

Figure 12.16 Oxidation of glucose

  ## Matching and colouring

83. Figure 12.17 summarizes the biochemical fates of the main energy sources in the central metabolic pathways, but only the pathways for glucose are complete. Using the labels given below, and by inserting arrows appropriately to indicate conversion of one substance to ánother, show how proteins and fats also contribute to energy production.

ADP × 4	H₂O
Amino acids	Acetyl coenzyme A
ATP × 4	CO₂
Ketone bodies	Pyruvic acid
Fatty acids	Oxaloacetic acid
Glycerol	

84. Colour the ATP produced in yellow and the metabolic water in blue.

85. Which substance is essential for the citric acid cycle and oxidative phosphorylation, but is unnecessary for glycolysis?

_____.

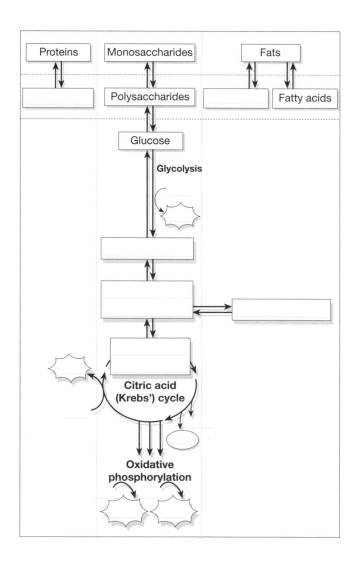

Figure 12.17 Summary of the central metabolic pathways

? MCQs

6. In the glomerulus, the efferent arteriole (choose all that apply): _____.

   a. Brings blood to the glomerular capsule
   b. Takes blood away from the glomerular capsule
   c. Is narrower than the afferent arteriole
   d. Is wider than the afferent arteriole.

7. The nephron includes the (choose all that apply): _____.

   a. Glomerulus   b. Proximal convoluted tubule   c. Distal convoluted tubule d. Medullary loop.

8. The principal effect of aldosterone is to increase reabsorption of: _____.

   a. Potassium   b. Calcium   c. Urea   d. Sodium.

9. Renin secretion is stimulated by (choose all that apply): _____.

   a. Low blood potassium   b. Low blood sodium   c. Low blood volume   d. Low blood pressure.

10. The proportion of glomerular filtrate reabsorbed is about: _____.

    a. 1%   b. 10%   c. 50%   d. 99%

11. The glomerular filtration rate (GFR) is normally about: _____.

    a. 8 litres per day   b. 90 litres per day   c. 180 litres per day   d. 900 litres per day.

  ## Colouring and completion

12. List the three processes involved in the formation of urine:

    - _____
    - _____
    - _____.

13. Colour the blood vessels on Figure 13.5.

14. Draw arrows on Fig. 13.5 to show the regions of the nephron where the processes listed above occur.

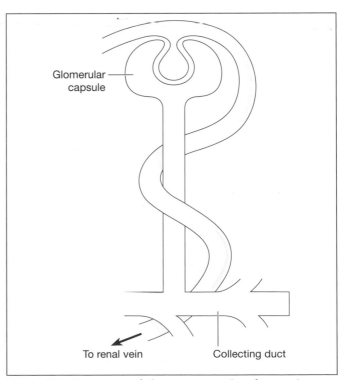

Figure 13.5 Summary of the processes that form urine

Completion

15. Complete Table 13.1 by identifying the characteristics of normal urine.

Colour	
Specific gravity	
pH	
Average daily volume	

Table 13.1 Characteristics of normal urine

16. Complete Table 13.2 by identifying which of the constituents of blood normally enter the glomerular filtrate and urine (insert 'normal' or 'abnormal' in each box).

Constituent of blood	Presence in glomerular filtrate	Presence in urine
Water		
Sodium		
Potassium		
Glucose		
Urea		
Creatinine		
Proteins		
Uric acid		
Red blood cells		
White blood cells		
Platelets		

Table 13.2 Normal constituents of glomerular filtrate and urine

17. Complete the blanks in the paragraph below to explain the control of water volume in the body.

Water is excreted through the lungs in _____, through the skin as _____ and via the kidneys as the main constituent of _____. Of these three, the most important in controlling fluid balance are the

_____. The minimum urinary output required to excrete the body's waste products is about

_____ per day. The volume in excess of this is controlled mainly by the hormone _____. Sensory

nerve cells, called _____, detect changes in the osmotic pressure of the blood. They are situated in the

_____. When the osmotic pressure increases, secretion of ADH is _____ and water is _____

by the distal collecting tubules and collecting ducts. These actions result in the osmotic pressure of the blood being

_____. This control system maintains osmotic pressure of the blood within a narrow

range and is known as a _____ system.

Matching

18. Figure 13.6 summarises the main processes involved in the renin-angiotensin-aldosterone system. Enter the appropriate letter from Figure 13.6 next to each of the key choices listed:

Key choices:

Sodium ____

Potassium ____

Water ____

Increased ____

Volume ____

Vasoconstriction ____

Renin ____

ACE (angiotensin converting enzyme) ____

Aldosterone ____.

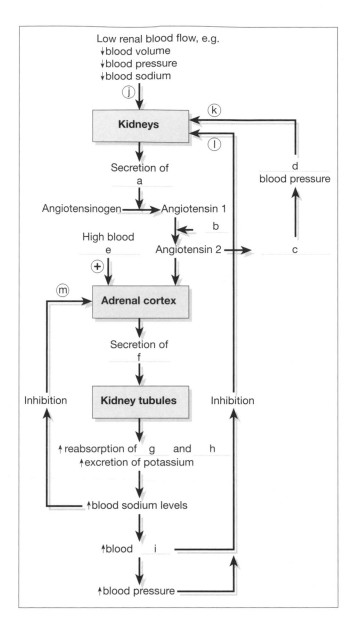

19. Add + or – beside the circles labelled j, k, l and m in Figure 13.6 to indicate whether the arrows stimulate or inhibit the feedback system.

Figure 13.6 Negative feedback regulation of aldosterone secretion

 ## Completion

20. Complete the second column of Table 13.3 by adding the site of production of each substance.

Substance	Site of production
Antidiuretic hormone	
Aldosterone	
Angiotensin converting enzyme	
Renin	
Angiotensinogen	
Atrial natriuretic peptide	

Table 13.3 The sites of production of substances that influence the composition of urine

URETERS

Completion

21. Fill in the blanks in the paragraph below to describe the structure of the ureters.

The ureters propel urine from the _____ to the bladder by the process of _____. Each ureter is about

_____ long and _____ in diameter. They enter the bladder at an _____ angle that prevents

_____ of urine into the ureter as the bladder fills and during _____.

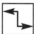 MCQs

22. The ureters are lined with: _____.

   a. Transitional epithelium   **b.** Stratified squamous epithelium   **c.** Ciliated columnar epithelium
   d. Pseudostratified epithelium.

23. Urine moves along the ureters by: _____.

   a. Gravity   **b.** Peristalsis   **c.** Active transport   **d.** Diffusion.

24. The ureters pass through the (choose all that apply):_____.

   a. Cranial cavity   **b.** Abdominal cavity   **c.** Pelvic cavity   **d.** Thoracic cavity.

25. The angle at which the ureters enter the bladder is: _____.

   a. Acute   **b.** Right   **c.** Square   **d.** Oblique.

URINARY BLADDER

Colouring and matching

26. Colour and match the following layers of the bladder with those shown on Figure 13.7:

○ Fibrous layer
○ Smooth muscle layer
○ Inner layer

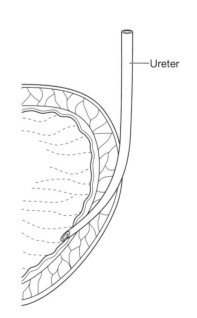

Ureter

Figure 13.7 The position of the ureter where it passes through the bladder wall

Colouring, matching and labelling

27. Colour and match the following structures on Figures 13.8A and B:

- ○ Rectum
- ○ Pubic bone
- ○ Anterior abdominal wall
- ○ Bladder
- ○ Right ureter

28. Colour and label the remaining structures on Figures 13.8A and B.

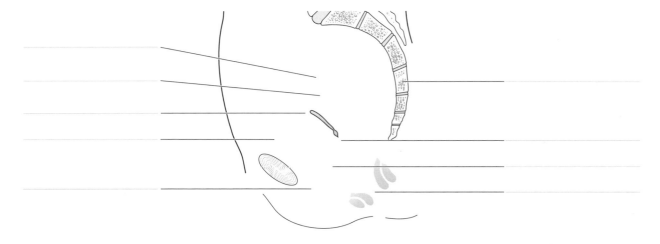

A   Female

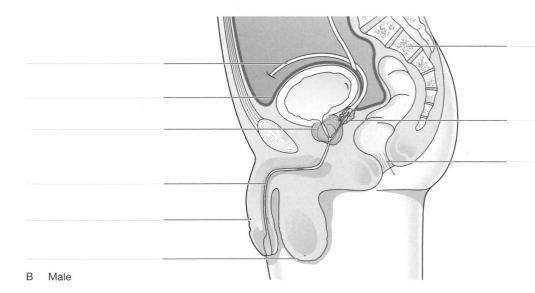

B   Male

Figure 13.8 Organs associated with the bladder in the male and female

✎ Completion

29. Fill in the blanks in the paragraph below describing the structure of the bladder.

The bladder acts as a _____ for urine. When empty, its shape resembles a _____ and it becomes more

_____ as it fills. The posterior surface is the _____ and the bladder opens into the urethra at its lowest point,

the _____. The bladder wall is composed of three layers. The outer layer is composed of _____ and

contains _____ and _____ vessels. The muscular layer is formed by _____ muscle arranged in

_____ layers. Collectively this is called the _____ and when it contracts the bladder _____. The inner

layer is the _____ and it is lined with _____. Three orifices on the posterior bladder wall form the

_____. The two upper openings are formed when each _____ enters the bladder and the lower one is

the opening of the _____.

URETHRA

❓ MCQs

30. The urethra extends from the: _____.

   a. Kidneys to the external urethral orifice
   b. Trigone to the external urethral orifice
   c. Base of the bladder to the external urethral orifice
   d. Neck of the bladder to the external urethral orifice.

31. How many layers of tissue are found in the wall of the urethra? _____.

   a. One   b. Two   c. Three   d. Four.

32. The internal urethral sphincter is composed of elastic tissue and: _____.

   a. Fibrous tissue   b. Smooth muscle   c. Skeletal muscle   d. Cardiac muscle.

33. The external urethral sphincter is composed of: _____.

   a. Fibrous tissue   b. Smooth muscle   c. Skeletal muscle   d. Cardiac muscle.

34. The urethra is (choose all that apply): _____.

   a. Part of the genital tract in males
   b. Part of the genital tract in females
   c. Longer in males than in females
   d. Longer in females than in males.

MICTURITION

 Matching

35. Select key choices from the list below to complete the blank spaces in the paragraph to describe the differences in micturition in infants and adults.

Key choices:

Brain	Over-ridden
Contraction	Relaxation
Detrusor	Spinal reflex
External	Stretching
Internal	Voluntary

As the bladder fills and becomes distended, receptors in the wall are stimulated by _____. In infants this

initiates a _____ and micturition occurs as nerve impulses to the bladder cause _____ of the

_____ muscle and _____ of the _____ urethral sphincter. When the nervous system is fully

developed the micturition reflex is stimulated but sensory impulses pass upwards to the _____. By conscious

effort, the reflex can be _____. In addition to the processes involved in infants, there is _____

relaxation of the _____ urethral sphincter.

Definitions

Define the following terms:

36. Polyuria _____

_____.

37. Glycosuria _____

_____.

38. Polydipsia _____

_____.

39. Ketonuria _____

_____.

✎ Applying what you know

40. In some kidney disorders the glomerular capillaries become more permeable. Substances that do not normally cross may then enter the filtrate and are excreted in the urine. Give three such examples.

- _____

- _____

- _____.

41. In diabetes mellitus raised blood sugar levels result in high concentrations of glucose in the glomerular filtrate. Explain the effects of this.

_____

_____

_____

_____

_____

42. In diabetes insipidus secretion of ADH is impaired. Describe the effects of this on urine output.

_____

_____

_____

43. ACE inhibitors are a group of drugs that inhibit the action of angiotensin converting enzyme. State their effects on blood pressure.

_____

_____

14 The skin

The skin completely covers the body and is continuous with the membranes that line the body orifices. This chapter will help you to learn about its structure and functions.

STRUCTURE OF THE SKIN

 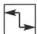 ### Colouring and labelling

1. Colour the capillaries on Figure 14.1.

2. Colour and label the structures identified on Figure 14.1.

3. Colour the following layers of the skin:

○ Epidermis   ○ Dermis   ○ Subcutaneous tissue

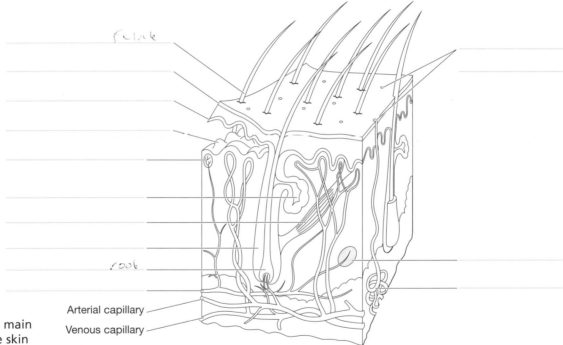

Figure 14.1 The main structures in the skin

Arterial capillary
Venous capillary

 ### MCQs

4. The healthy epidermis is formed by: _____.

   a. One thick layer of columnar epithelium
   b. Several layers of connective tissue
   c. Division of epithelial cells in the basal layer that are pushed upwards
   d. Blood vessels, nerve endings, sebaceous glands and sweat glands.

5. Complete regeneration of the epidermis takes about: _____.

   a. 1 day   **b.** 7 days   **c.** 28 days   **d.** 120 days.

6. Keratin is found in (choose all that apply): _____.

   a. Hair   **b.** Nails   **c.** Sweat glands   **d.** Epidermis.

7. Melanin is a (choose all that apply): _____.

   a. Neurotransmitter present in sensory nerve endings
   b. Coloured pigment formed from the amino acid tyrosine
   c. Constituent of sebum secreted by the sebaceous glands
   d. Substance that protects the skin from harmful effects of sunlight.

Completion

8. Complete Table 14.1 by inserting the stimulus to each of the receptors found in the skin.

Sensory receptor	Stimulus
Meissner's corpuscle	
Pacinian corpuscle	
Free nerve ending	

Table 14.1 Sensory receptors and their stimuli

FUNCTIONS OF THE SKIN

Matching

9. Match the correct key choice with the appropriate statement.

   Key choices:

   Langerhans cells   Vasodilation

   Sensory nerve endings   Non-specific defence mechanism

   Conduction   Absorption

   Evaporation   Vitamin D

   Convection

   a. Stimulation may initiate a reflex response: _____

   b. Occurs when objects in contact with the skin take up heat: _____

   c. Results in increased blood flow and is recognized by redness of the skin: _____

   d. Formed by conversion of 7-dehydrocholesterol by UV rays in sunlight: _____

   e. Specialized immune cells: _____

   f. Takes place when heat is used to convert water in sweat to water vapour: _____

   g. The mechanism by which a limited number of substances gain entry to the body: _____

   h. Occurs as cool air replaces warmed air which has risen from the body: _____

   i. A means of protection against many different potential dangers: _____.

? Pot luck

10. State whether each process results in heat loss or heat gain.

a. Shivering _____

b. Sweating _____

c. Conduction _____

d. Radiation _____

e. Vasodilation _____

f. Vasoconstriction _____

g. Evaporation _____

h. Convection _____ .

✎ Completion

11. Fill in the blanks to complete the paragraphs describing temperature regulation.

The temperature regulating centre is situated in the _____ and is responsive to the

temperature of circulating _____. When body temperature rises, sweat glands are stimulated by the

_____. The _____ centre in the medulla oblongata controls the diameter of small

arteries and _____ and therefore the amount of _____ circulating in the dermis. When body

temperature rises the skin capillaries _____ and extra blood near the surface increases heat loss by

_____, _____ and _____. The skin is warm and _____ in colour. When body temperature

falls, arteriolar vasoconstriction conserves heat and the skin is _____ and feels cool.

Fever is often the result of _____. During this process there is release of chemicals, also called

_____, from damaged tissue. These chemicals act on the _____ which releases prostaglandins

that reset the temperature thermostat to a _____ temperature. The body responds by activating heat

promoting mechanisms, e.g. _____ and _____, until the new temperature is reached. When

the thermostat is reset to the normal level, heat loss mechanisms are activated. There is vasodilatation and profuse

_____ until body temperature returns to the normal range again.

WOUND HEALING

 Completion

12. Complete Table 14.2 by identifying factors that affect the rate of wound healing.

	Promote wound healing	Impair wound healing
Systemic factors	_____ _____	_____ _____
Local factors	_____	_____

Table 14.2 Factors affecting the rate of wound healing

 Definitions

Define the following terms:

13. Primary healing _____.

14. Secondary healing _____.

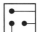 **Colouring and labelling**

15. Identify the stages of wound healing shown in Figure 14.2.

16. Colour the following on Figure 14.2:

○ Fibroblasts
○ Phagocytes

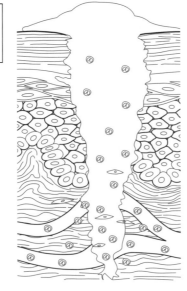 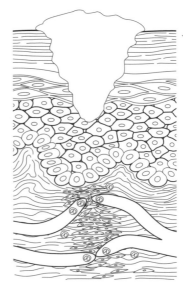 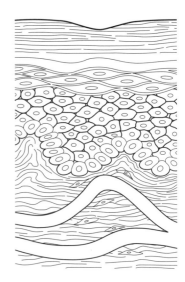

Figure 14.2 Stages in primary wound healing

? MCQs

17. In wound healing, phagocytes (choose all that apply): _____.

    a. Secrete collagen fibres
    b. Remove clotted blood and debris by phagocytosis
    c. Travel to the wound in its blood supply
    d. Form the scab that separates after 3–10 days.

18. In wound healing, fibroblasts (choose all that apply): _____.

    a. Secrete collagen fibres
    b. Remove clotted blood and debris by phagocytosis
    c. Travel to the wound in its blood supply
    d. Form the scab that separates after 3–10 days.

19. Granulation tissue (choose all that apply): _____.

    a. Is formed during primary healing
    b. Is formed during secondary healing
    c. Is another term for scar tissue
    d. Consists of capillary buds, phagocytes and fibroblasts.

20. Slough is: _____.

    a. Healthy tissue
    b. Necrotic tissue
    c. A substance that promotes wound healing
    d. Another term for granulation tissue.

21. Scar tissue (choose all that apply): _____.

    a. Is shiny
    b. Contains sweat glands and hair follicles
    c. Is formed from granulation tissue
    d. Is formed from fibrous tissue.

✐ Applying what you know

22. Define the term hypothermia _____
    _____.

23. Outline why the skin is pale in hypothermia _____
    _____.

24. Explain why shivering starts and stops again as core body temperature decreases
    _____
    _____
    _____.

15 Resistance and immunity

From life in the womb to the moment of death, an individual is under constant attack from an enormous range of potentially harmful invaders, including bacteria, viruses, parasites and foreign (non-self) cells. The body has therefore developed a wide range of protective measures, both specific and non-specific, which will be considered in this chapter.

Definitions

Define the following terms:

1. Non-specific resistance _____

    _____

    _____.

2. Specific resistance _____

    _____.

NON-SPECIFIC DEFENCE MECHANISMS

MCQs

3. Complement is (choose all that apply): _____.

    a. A system of about 20 antibodies found in the blood and body fluids
    b. Active against bacteria
    c. An effective attractant for white blood cells
    d. Produced by virally infected cells.

4. Which of the following induces resistance to viral infection? _____.

    a. Interleukin   **b.** Complement   **c.** Interferon   **d.** Lysozyme.

5. Which of the following is involved in specific defence? _____.

    a. Antibody   **b.** Interferon   **c.** Interleukin   **d.** Histamine.

6. Which of the following binds to, and perforates, bacterial cell walls? _____.

    a. Interferon   **b.** Histamine   **c.** Lysozyme   **d.** Complement.

Colouring and labelling

7. Which defensive process is shown in Figure 15.1?
   _____

8. Label the structures shown on Figure 15.1.

9. Briefly describe the events being shown in each part of Figure 15.1.

   a. _____

   b. _____

   c. _____

   d. _____

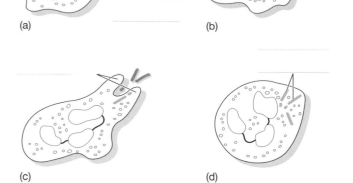

(a)   (b)

(c)   (d)

Figure 15.1 Action of neutrophils

Colouring, matching and labelling

10. Figure 15.2 summarizes the main events of the acute inflammatory reaction. Colour, match and identify the cells labelled A, B, C and D and their functions.

   ○ A _____
   _____

   ○ B _____
   _____

   ○ C _____
   _____

   ○ D _____
   _____.

11. Figure 15.2 shows three different inflammatory mediators. Identify them according to the information given by colouring and matching the symbols in the key.

   ○ Stored in preformed granules by cell C
   _____

   ※ Causes pain by acting on free nerve endings
   _____

   ⬡ Family of mediators made from cell membranes
   _____.

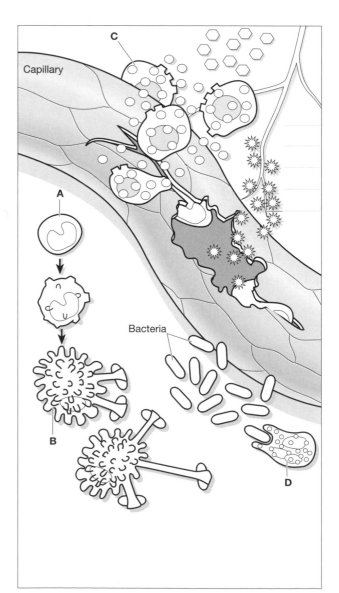

Figure 15.2 The inflammatory response

? | Pot luck

12. List the five main signs of the inflammatory response:

- _____
- _____
- _____
- _____
- _____

? | MCQs

13. Increased blood flow to an inflamed area is due to: _____.

a. Attraction of large numbers of white blood cells into the region
b. Loss of plasma proteins from the bloodstream
c. Dilation of blood vessels supplying the area
d. Increased vascular permeability, caused by histamine.

14. The predominant white blood cell in the early inflammatory response is the: _____.

a. Monocyte   **b.** Macrophage   **c.** Eosinophil   **d.** Neutrophil.

15. Chemotaxis is (choose all that apply): _____.

a. Movement of white blood cells out of the bloodstream into the tissues
b. Attraction of white blood cells to an area of inflammation
c. Stimulated by substances released from white blood cells
d. Seen only in the early stages of an acute inflammatory response.

16. An inflamed area swells because (choose all that apply): _____.

a. Blood supply to the area increases
b. Blood vessels in the region become more permeable
c. There is loss of plasma proteins from the bloodstream
d. Hydrostatic pressure within local blood vessels increases.

Completion

17. Table 15.1 lists some important information about significant inflammatory mediators. Complete the table by filling in the blanks.

Substance	Made by	Trigger for release	Main actions
Histamine			
	Platelets, mast cells and basophils; neurotransmitter in central nervous system		
	Synthesized as required from cell membranes		
			Anticoagulant, maintaining blood supply to an inflamed area
Bradykinin			

Table 15.1 Summary of some important inflammatory mediators

? **MCQs**

18. Raised temperature, both local and systemic, is beneficial in the inflammatory response because it (choose all that apply): _____.

    a. Enhances phagocytosis   **c.** Decreases bacterial viability
    b. Increases chemotaxis   **d.** Increases production of prostaglandins and other inflammatory mediators.

19. Which plasma protein leaks into the tissues and forms an insoluble barrier around an infected area? _____.

    a. Thromboplastin   **b.** Fibrinogen   **c.** Plasmin   **d.** Albumin.

20. Which mediator is responsible for resetting the internal thermostat in the hypothalamus in infection, leading to fever? _____.

    a. Prostaglandin E_2 **b.** Bradykinin   **c.** Interferon   **d.** Interleukin 1.

21. Which type of white blood cell predominates in chronic inflammation? _____.

    a. Lymphocytes   **b.** Macrophages   **c.** Neutrophils   **d.** Eosinophils.

22. Immunological surveillance is:

    a. Mediated by macrophages   **c.** An essential part of the acute inflammatory response
    b. Ineffective against virally infected cells   **d.** Important in the detection of mutated body cells

IMMUNITY

 Completion

23. Table 15.2 lists various characteristics of the two main populations of lymphocyte. Complete the table.

Characteristic	T-lymphocyte	B-lymphocyte
Shape of nucleus		
Site of manufacture		
Site of post-manufacture processing		
Nature of immunity involved		
Specific or non-specific defence		
Production of antibodies		
Processing regulated by thymosin		

Table 15.2 Lymphocyte characteristics

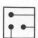 **Matching, labelling and colouring**

24. Figure 15.3 shows how the production of the different types of T-lymphocyte comes about. Identify the different types of cell and the function of each using the key below.

   O Macrophage

   Function: _____

   O T-lymphocyte, unspecialized

   Function: _____

   O Cytotoxic T-lymphocyte

   Function: _____

   O Helper T-lymphocyte

   Function: _____

   O Memory T-lymphocyte

   Function: _____

   O Suppressor T-lymphocyte

   Function: _____

25. Label the remaining items indicated on Figure 15.3.

26. Colour the receptors for antigen on all cells you see.
   What is significant about these receptors when you compare them between cell types?

   _____

   _____

27. The process of proliferation and differentiation shown in the centre of the diagram is also known as what?

   _____

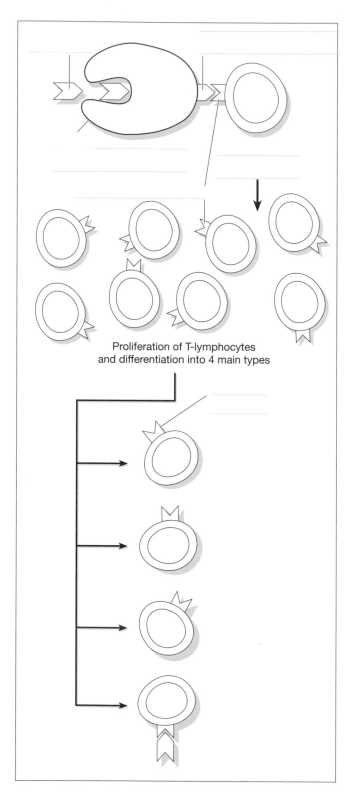

Proliferation of T-lymphocytes and differentiation into 4 main types

Figure 15.3 Production of subtypes of T-lymphocytes

Matching, labelling and colouring

28. Figure 15.4 shows how the production of the different types of B-lymphocyte comes about. Colour and match the different types of cell and the function of each using the key below.

○ Helper T-lymphocyte

Function: _____

○ B-lymphocyte

Function: _____

○ Memory B-lymphocyte

Function: _____

○ Plasma cell

Function: _____

29. Label the remaining items indicated on Figure 15.4.

30. Explain what is represented at A in Figure 15.4.

_____

_____

31. Colour the receptors for antigen on any cell you see. What is significant about these receptors when you compare them between cell types?

_____

_____

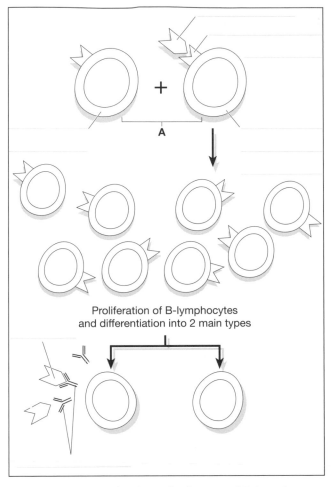

Proliferation of B-lymphocytes and differentiation into 2 main types

Figure 15.4 Production of subtypes of B-lymphocytes

? MCQs

32. Which of the cell types in Figure 15.3 is important in both cell-mediated and antibody-mediated immunity? ___.

  a. Macrophage   **b.** Cytotoxic T-lymphocyte   **c.** Helper T-lymphocyte   **d.** Memory T-lymphocyte.

33. Which of the cell types in Figure 15.3 is longest lived? _____.

  a. Macrophage   **b.** Cytotoxic T-lymphocyte   **c.** Helper T-lymphocyte   **d.** Memory T-lymphocyte.

34. Which of the cell types in Figure 15.3 is active against different types of antigen (i.e. it is not specific)? _____.

  a. Macrophage   **b.** Cytotoxic T-lymphocyte   **c.** Helper T-lymphocyte   **d.** Memory T-lymphocyte.

35. What is the expected life span of a plasma cell? _____.

  a. The individual's lifetime   **b.** A year or more   **c.** A month or so   **d.** No more than a day.

Completion

36. The following paragraph discusses the antibody response to antigen exposure. Complete it by filling in the blanks.

When the body is exposed to an antigen for the first time, the immune response can be measured as antibody

levels in the blood after about _____ weeks; this is the _____ response. Antibody levels fall thereafter,

and do not rise again unless there is a second exposure to the same antigen, which stimulates a _____

response, which is different from the first in that it is much _____ and antibody levels become much

_____. After having been exposed to an antigen, an individual may develop immunity to it, provided he has

produced a population of _____ cells.

37. Immunity may be acquired in different ways, and the nature of the immunity may vary. Complete Table 15.3 by ticking the appropriate boxes relevant to each of the four listed types of immunity.

Characteristic	Active natural	Active artificial	Passive natural	Passive artificial
An example is a baby's consumption of antibodies in its mother's milk				
Long-lived protection				
Involves production of memory cells				
An example is vaccination				
Short-lived protection				
An example is infusion of antibodies				
Involves production of antibodies by the individual				
An example is a child catching chickenpox at school				
Specific				

Table 15.3 The four types of acquired immunity

16 The musculoskeletal system

The musculoskeletal system consists of the bones of the skeleton, their joints and the skeletal (voluntary) muscles that move the body. This chapter will help you to understand the structure and function of each component of the musculoskeletal system.

BONE

 Colouring and matching

1. Colour and match the following parts of the long bone on Figure 16.1:

- ○ Compact bone
- ○ Spongy bone
- ○ Medullary canal
- ○ Nutrient artery
- ○ Articular cartilage
- ○ Epiphyseal plate

2. Name the vascular membrane that covers bone:

_____.

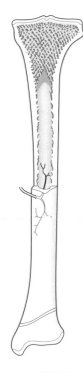

Figure 16.1 A mature long bone – partially sectioned

Completion

3. Give an example of each type of bone:

a. Long _____

b. Short _____

c. Irregular _____

d. Flat _____

e. Sesamoid _____.

Labelling

4. In Figure 16.2, which shows the microscopic structure of compact bone, label the parts indicated.

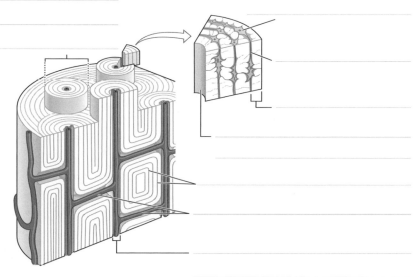

Figure 16.2 Microscopic structure of compact bone

Matching

5. Match the key choices with the statements in Table 16.1.

Key choices:

Sesamoid bones

Flat bones

Long bones

Chondroblasts

Lacunae

Osteon

Osteoblasts

Osteoclasts

Osteocytes

Red bone marrow

Trabeculae

Interstitial lamellae

Spongy bone

Spongy bone

Cortical bone.

Table 16.1 Characteristics of bone

	Looks like a honeycomb to the naked eye
	Cells that lay down bone
	Cells that break down bone
	Haversian system
	Cancellous bone
	Compact bone
	Form the framework of spongy bone
	Cells that lay down cartilage
	Mature osteoblasts
	Remains of old osteons
	Spaces between lamellae that contain osteocytes
	Found mainly in spaces within spongy bone
	Develop from membrane models
	Develop from tendon models
	Develop from cartilage models

 Completion

6. To make the following paragraph read correctly, delete the incorrect options in bold. Take care, there may be more than one correct answer in each set of options!

Bone tissue develops in the foetus from **adipose/connective/epithelial tissue** models. This process is called

osteogenesis/oogenesis/ossification and is **usually complete/incomplete/always complete** at birth. The main

constituent of bone is **water/calcium salts/bone marrow**, and the organic component is primarily

cartilage/phosphate/collagen. During life, bone growth is stimulated by **parathormone/thyroxine/oestrogen**,

but its density is decreased by **calcium/testosterone/lack of exercise**.

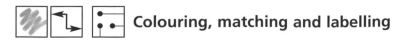 **Colouring, matching and labelling**

17. Colour and match the following skull bones shown
on Figure 16.4:

○ Ethmoid bone

○ Frontal bone

○ Lacrimal bone

○ Occipital bone

○ Maxilla

○ Mandible

○ Nasal bone

○ Parietal bone

○ Sphenoid bone

○ Temporal bone

○ Zygomatic bone

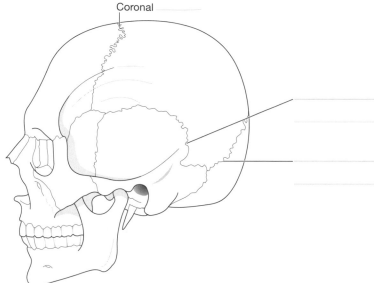

Coronal

Figure 16.4 The bones of the skull and their sutures

18. Label the skull sutures identified on Figure 16.4.

 Completion

19. State which bone(s) of the skull:

    a. Form(s) the posterior part of the hard palate: _____

    b. Form(s) the anterior part of the hard palate: _____

    c. Form(s) the main part of the nasal septum: _____

    d. Form(s) the most posterior part: _____

    e. Give(s) rise to the mastoid processes: _____

    f. Contain(s) the hypophyseal fossa: _____

    g. Form(s) the cribriform plate: _____

    h. Contain(s) the middle ear: _____

    i. Contain(s) the foramen magnum: _____

    j. Contain(s) the foramina for the nasolacrimal ducts: _____.

20. Fill in the blanks to complete the description of sinuses and fontanelles of the skull.

Sinuses contain _____ and are found in the _____, _____, _____ and _____

bones. They all communicate with the _____ and are lined with _____. Their

functions are to give _____ to the voice and_____ the bones of the face and cranium.

   Fontanelles are distinct _____ areas of the skull in infants and are present until _____ is

complete and the skull bones fuse. The largest are the _____ fontanelle, present until _____ months,

and the _____ fontanelle that usually closes over by _____ months of age. Their presence allows for

moulding of the baby's _____ during childbirth.

Colouring and matching

21. Colour and match the following parts of Figure 16.5:

- ○ Intervertebral discs
- ○ Cervical vertebrae
- ○ Thoracic vertebrae
- ○ Lumbar vertebrae
- ○ Sacrum
- ○ Coccyx

22. State the number of:

   a. Cervical vertebrae _____

   b. Thoracic vertebrae _____

   c. Lumbar vertebrae _____

   d. Vertebrae that fuse to form the sacrum _____

   e. Vertebrae that fuse to form the coccyx _____.

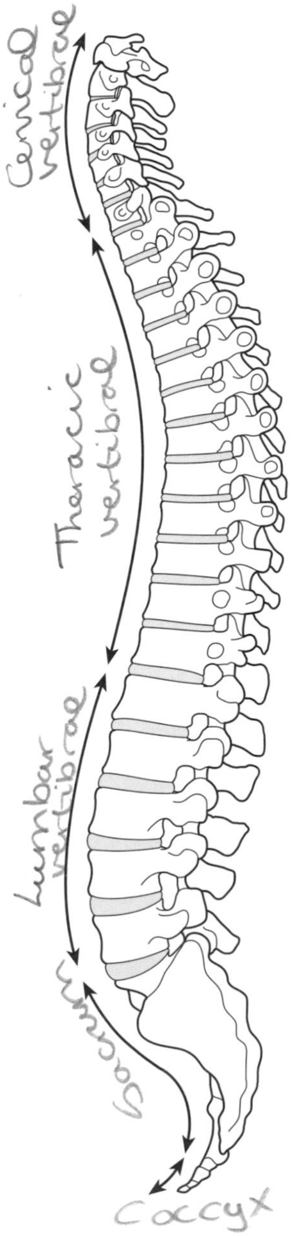

Figure 16.5 The vertebral column. Lateral view

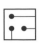 **Labelling and matching**

23. Match and label the parts of a typical vertebra shown in Figure 16.6:

Body
Lamina
Pedicle
Spinous process
Superior articular process
Transverse process
Vertebral foramen

Anterior aspect

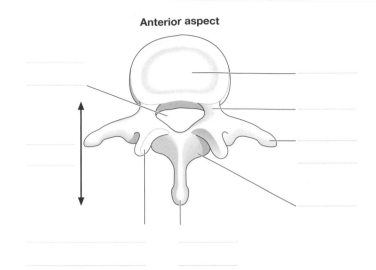

Figure 16.6 A lumbar vertebra showing features of a typical vertebra, viewed from above

 Matching

24. Match the key choices listed with the statements about the vertebral column below:

Key choices:

Odontoid process

Intervertebral disc

Sacrum

Axis

Thoracic vertebrae

Vertebral foramen

Nucleus pulposus

Atlas

Coccyx

Annulus fibrosus

Transverse foramen

a. Consists of four fused vertebrae: _____

b. Part of a cervical vertebra containing the vertebral artery:_____

c. Vertebrae that articulate with ribs: _____

d. First cervical vertebra: _____

e. Second cervical vertebra: _____

f. Articulates with the ilium to form the sacroiliac joints _____

g. Acts as the body of the atlas: _____

h. Part of the vertebrae containing the spinal cord: _____

i. Separates the bodies of adjacent vertebrae: _____

j. The outer part of the intervertebral disc: _____

k. The central core of the intervertebral disc: _____.

Colouring and matching

25. Colour and match the following structures shown in Figure 16.7:

○ Costal cartilages
○ Ribs attached to sternum
○ Floating ribs
○ Sternum
○ Clavicles
○ Vertebrae

26. Name the nerves running in the groove found on the underside of each rib _____.

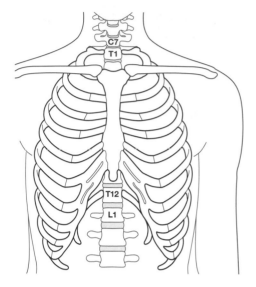

Figure 16.7 The thoracic cage. Anterior view

APPENDICULAR SKELETON

  Matching and labelling

27. Label Figure 16.8 to show the parts of the scapula using the list below.

Parts of the scapula

Acromion process

Coracoid process

Glenoid cavity

Inferior angle

Infraspinous fossa

Lateral border

Medial border

Spine

Supraspinous fossa

Superior angle

Superior border

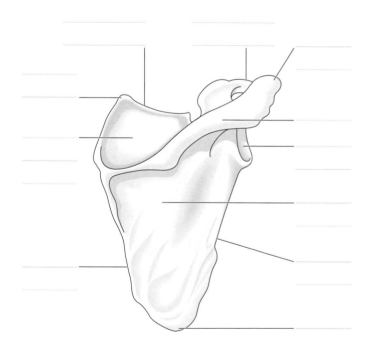

Figure 16.8 The right scapula. Posterior view

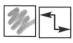 **Colouring, matching and labelling**

28. Match and label the parts of the humerus on Figure 16.9 using the terms listed below.

Parts of the humerus

Head

Neck

Shaft

Greater tubercle

Lesser tubercle

Bicipital groove

Capitulum

Coronoid fossa

Deltoid tuberosity

Lateral supracondylar ridge

Medial supracondylar ridge

Lateral epicondyle

Medial epicondyle

Trochlea

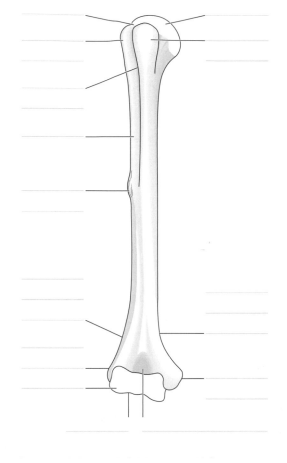

Figure 16.9 The right humerus. Anterior view

29. On Figure 16.10, colour and match the following:

- ○ Radius
- ○ Ulna
- ○ Olecranon process
- ○ Interosseus membrane

30. Identify and label the structures shown on Figure 16.10.

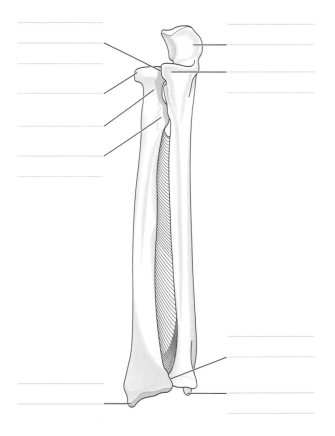

Figure 16.10 The right radius and ulna

31. Colour and match the following parts of Figure 16.11:

○ The carpal bones
○ The metacarpal bones
○ The proximal phalanges
○ The middle phalanges
○ The distal phalanges

32. Name the bones of the wrist shown on Figure 16.11.

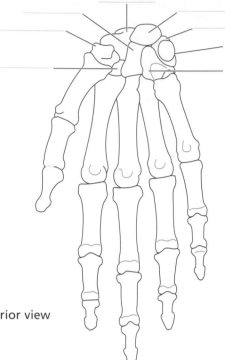

Figure 16.11 The bones of the wrist, hand and fingers. Anterior view

 Pot luck

33. Name the bone on which the following landmarks are found:

a. Deltoid tuberosity: _____   **c.** Olecranon process: _____

b. Acromion process: _____   **d.** Glenoid cavity: _____.

  Colouring, matching and labelling

34. On Figure 16.12, colour and match the three fused bones that form the hip bone:

○ Ilium
○ Ischium
○ Pubis

35. Identify the bony landmarks of the hip bone indicated on Figure 16.12.

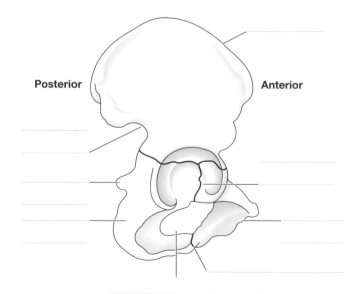

Posterior   Anterior

Figure 16.12 The right hip bone. Lateral view

36. On Figure 16.13, colour and match the following parts of the femur:

○ Neck
○ Head
○ Shaft

37. Label the landmarks of the femur indicated on Figure 16.13.

38. On Figure 16.14, colour and match the following parts of the lower limb:

○ Tibia
○ Fibula
○ Interosseus membrane

39. Label the bony landmarks identified on Figure 16.14.

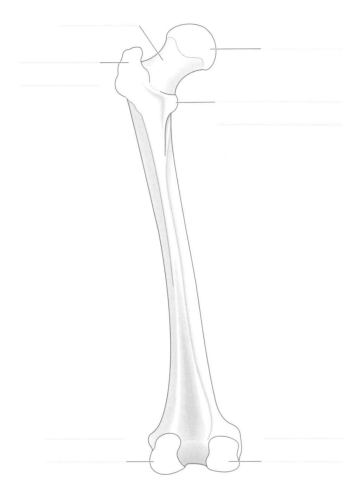

Figure 16.13 The left femur. Posterior view

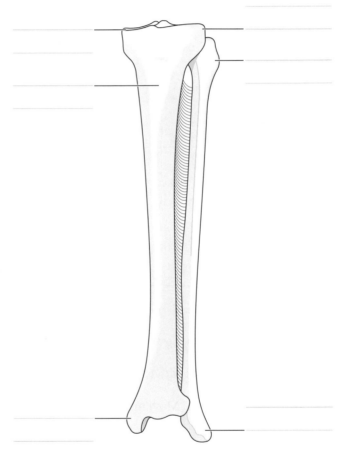

Figure 16.14 The left tibia and fibula. Anterior view

40. What is the function of the interosseous membrane? _____

_____

41. On Figure 16.15, colour and match the following parts of the foot:

○ Tarsal bones
○ Metatarsal bones
○ Phalanges

42. Label the tarsal bones of the foot shown on Figure 16.15.

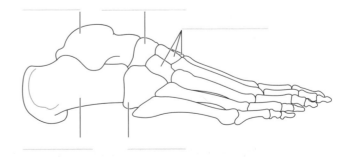

Figure 16.15 The bones of the foot. Lateral view

JOINTS

 Completion

43. Complete the blank columns in Table 16.3 by naming the type of joint listed, using S=synovial, F=fibrous or C=cartilaginous, and identifying the range of movement possible at that joint using I=immovable, Sl=slightly movable and Fr=freely movable.

	Type (S, F or C)	Movement (I, Sl, Fr)
Suture		
Tooth in jaw		
Shoulder joint		
Symphysis pubis		
Knee joint		
Interosseous membrane		
Hip joint		
Joint between phalanges		
Intervertebral discs		

Table 16.3 Joints and movements.

Matching

44. Match the key choices to define the movements listed below.

Key choices:

Abduction

Adduction

Circumduction

Eversion

Extension

Flexion

Inversion

Pronation

Rotation

Supination

a. Bending, usually forwards: _____

b. Straightening or bending backwards: _____

c. Movement away from the midline of the body: _____

d. Movement towards the midline of the body: _____

e. Movement of a limb or digit so that it forms a cone in space: _____

f. Movement round the long axis of a bone: _____

g. Turning the palm of the hand down: _____

h. Turning the palm of the hand up: _____

i. Turning the sole of the foot inwards: _____

j. Turning the sole of the foot outwards: _____.

Colouring and labelling

45. Colour and label the following parts of the
synovial joint on Figure 16.16:

Bone
Capsular ligament
Synovial membrane
Articular cartilage
Synovial cavity

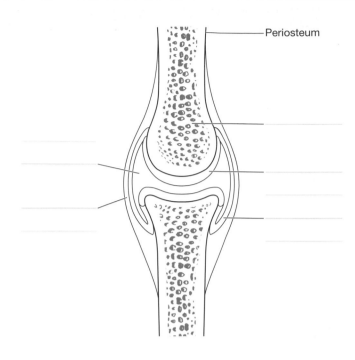

Periosteum

Figure 16.16 The basic structure of a synovial joint

? **Pot luck**

46. List three functions of synovial fluid:

- _____

- _____

- _____.

47. State the function of the following extracapsular structures:

a. Ligaments: _____

_____

b. Muscles or their tendons: _____

_____.

MAIN SYNOVIAL JOINTS OF THE LIMBS

   Colouring, matching and labelling

48. Colour and match the following parts of the shoulder joint on Figure 16.17:

○ Capsular ligament
○ Synovial membrane
○ Articular cartilage
○ Synovial cavity

49. Label the parts of the shoulder indicated on Figure 16.17.

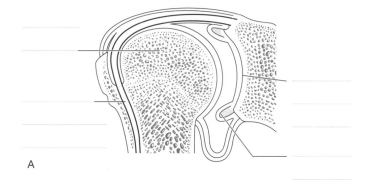

A

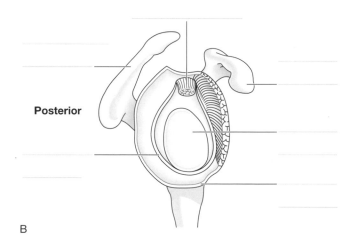

Posterior

B

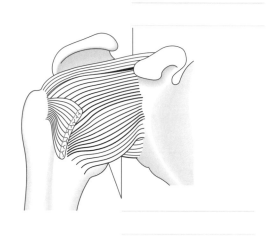

C

Figure 16.17 The right shoulder joint. A. Section viewed from the front. B. The position of the glenoidal labrum with the humerus removed. C. The supporting ligaments viewed from the front.

50. What type of synovial joint is the shoulder joint? _____

Completion

51. Identify the muscles, or combinations of muscles, involved in movements at the shoulder joint and complete Table 16.4.

Movement	Muscle(s) involved
Flexion	
Extension	
Abduction	
Adduction	
Circumduction	
Medial rotation	
Lateral rotation	

Table 16.4 Muscles involved in movement at the shoulder joint

52. What type of synovial joint is found at the elbow ? _____

53. Complete Table 16.5 by inserting the two types of movement possible at the elbow in the left-hand column and the muscles involved in the right hand column.

Movement	Muscle(s) involved

Table 16.5 Muscles involved in movement of the elbow

54. What type of synovial joint is found between the phalanges? _____

Matching

55. Insert the movements from the list of key choices to complete Table 16.6. (Take care, as you will not need all the key choices.)

Key choices:

Abduction

Adduction

Circumduction

Eversion

Extension

Flexion

Inversion

Pronation

Rotation

Supination

Movement of radioulnar joints	Muscle(s) involved
	Pronator teres
	Supinator, biceps
Movement of the wrist	
	Flexor carpi radialis, flexor carpi ulnaris
	Extensor carpi radialis (longis and brevis), extensor carpi ulnaris
	Flexor and extensor carpi radialis
	Flexor and extensor carpi ulnaris

Table 16.6 Muscles involved in movement of the proximal and distal radioulnar joints and wrist

56. What kind of synovial joint is found at the hip? _____

  Colouring, labelling and matching

57. Colour and match the following parts of the hip joint:

○ Capsular ligament

○ Synovial membrane

○ Articular cartilage

○ Synovial cavity

58. Label the parts of the hip joint indicated in Figure 16.18.

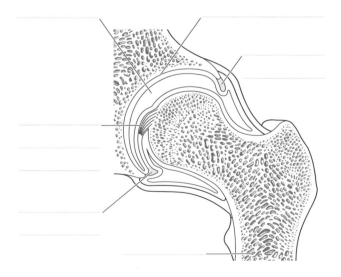

Figure 16.18 Section of the hip joint (anterior view)

Completion

59. Match the groups of muscles in the key choices below with the movements of the hip shown in Table 16.7:

Key choices:

Mainly gluteal muscles and adductor group

Gluteus medius and minimus, sartorius

Adductor group

Gluteus medius and minimus

Psoas, iliacus, rectus femoris, sartorius

Gluteus maximus, hamstrings

Table 16.7 Muscles involved in movement of the hip

Movement	Muscle(s) involved
Flexion	
Extension	
Abduction	
Adduction	
Medial rotation	
Lateral rotation	

   Colouring, matching and labelling

60. Colour and match the following structures of the knee joint on Figure 16.19A and B:

- ○ Articular cartilage
- ○ Capsular ligament
- ○ Cruciate ligament
- ○ Femur
- ○ Fibula
- ○ Patella
- ○ Synovial membrane
- ○ Semilunar cartilages
- ○ Tibia

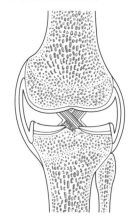

A

61. Label the remaining structures shown on Figure 16.19.

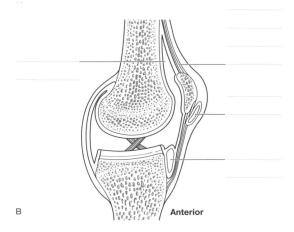

B

Anterior

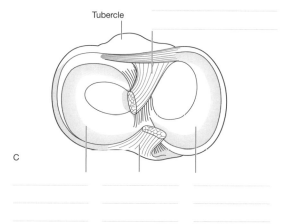

Tubercle

C

Figure 16.19 The knee joint. A. Section viewed from the front. B. Section viewed from the side. C. The superior surface of the tibia showing the semilunar cartilages and the cruciate ligaments

62. What kind of synovial joint is found at the knee? _____

Completion

63. Insert the key choices below to complete Table 16.8.

Key choices:

Hamstrings

Quadriceps femoris

Flexion

Gastrocnemius

Extension

Movement	Muscle(s) involved

Table 16.8 Muscles involved in movement of the knee

MUSCLE TISSUE

64. Name the three types of muscle:

- _____

- _____

- _____.

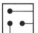 **Colouring and labelling**

65. Colour and label the parts of the skeletal muscle identified on Figure 16.20.

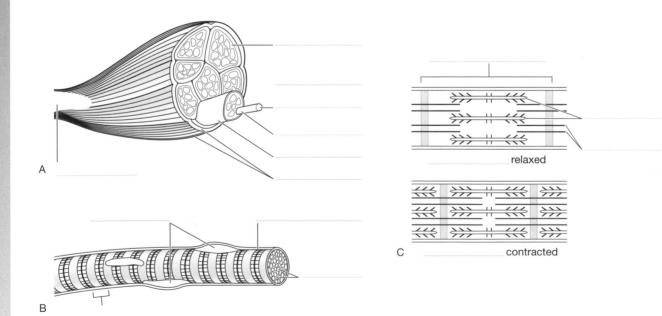

Figure 16.20 Organisation within a skeletal muscle

Completion

66. The following paragraph describes the sliding filament theory. Complete it by filling in the blanks.

The functional unit of a skeletal muscle cell is the _____. At each end of this unit are lines called ___-lines. Within the unit are two types of filament, thick filaments (made of _____), and thin ones, made of _____. When the muscle cell is relaxed, these two filaments are not connected to each other. Contraction is initiated when an electrical impulse, called an _____, passes along the cell membrane (also called the _____) of the muscle cell and penetrates deep into the sarcoplasm via the network of _____ that run through the cell. This electrical stimulation causes _____ ions to be released from the _____ within the cell; these ions cause links, called _____ to form between the thick and thin filaments. The filaments pull on each other, which causes the functional unit to _____ in length, pulling the _____ at either end towards one another. If enough units are stimulated to contract at the same time, the entire _____ will also _____.

? **Pot luck**

67. There are four errors in the paragraph below, which describes the neuromuscular junction. Find them and correct them.

The axons of sensory neurones conveying impulses to skeletal muscles divide into fine filaments that end in motor units. Each muscle fibre is stimulated at many motor end-plates and one motor nerve has many motor end-plates.

The nerve impulse is passed across the neuromuscular junction – the gap between the motor end-plate and the muscle fibre – by the neurotransmitter dopamine. The group of muscle fibres and the motor end-plates of the nerve fibres that supply them form a motor unit.

Labelling

68. Label the parts of the motor unit shown on Figure 16.21.

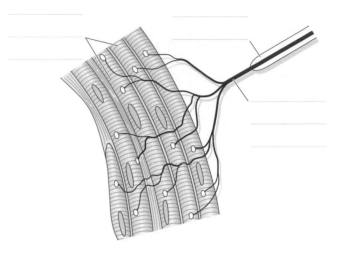

Figure 16.21 The neuromuscular junction

 Definitions

Define the terms:

69. Isotonic contraction _____

_____

70. Isometric contraction _____

_____

71. The origin of a muscle _____

_____

72. Hypertrophy of muscle _____

_____

73. Antagonistic pair _____

_____ .

MUSCLES OF THE FACE AND NECK

  Colouring and labelling

74. Colour and label the muscles shown in Figure 16.22.

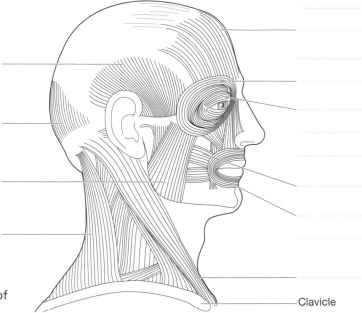

Figure 16.22 The main muscles on the right side of the face, head and neck

Clavicle

 Completion

75. Complete Table 16.9 to outline the functions of the muscles of the face and neck.

Muscle	Paired/unpaired	Function
Occipitofrontalis		
Levator palpebrae superioris		
Orbicularis oculi		
Buccinator		
Orbicularis oris		
Masseter		
Temporalis		
Pterygoid		
Sternocleidomastoid		Contraction of one side: Contraction of both sides:
Trapezius		

Table 16.9 Functions of muscles of the face and neck

MUSCLES OF THE BACK

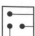 **Labelling**

76. Label the muscles of the back shown on Figure 16.23.

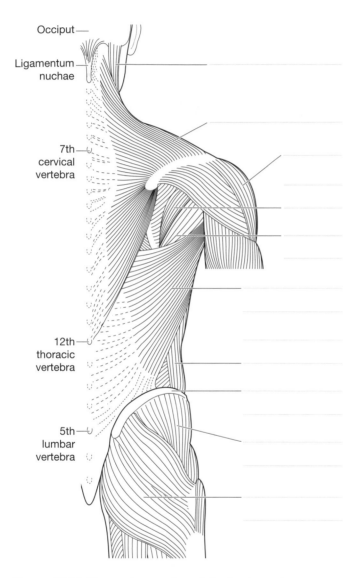

Occiput —

Ligamentum nuchae —

7th cervical vertebra —

12th thoracic vertebra —

5th lumbar vertebra —

Figure 16.23 The main muscles of the back

Figure 16.24 Transverse sections of the muscles and fasciae of the abdominal wall. A. Anterior wall. B. Posterior wall: a lumbar vertebra and its associated muscles

MUSCLES OF THE ABDOMINAL WALL

  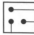 **Colouring, matching and labelling**

77. Colour and match these muscles on Figures 16.24A and B:

○ Internal oblique

○ External oblique.

○ Transversus abdominis

78. Colour and label the other structures shown on Figure 16.24.

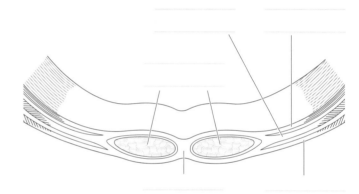

A

Anterior aspect

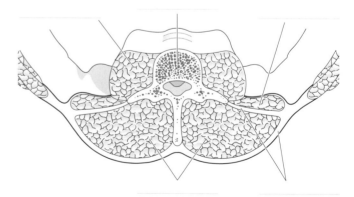

B

MUSCLES OF THE UPPER LIMBS

  Colouring and labelling

79. Colour and label the muscles of the upper limb on Figure 16.25

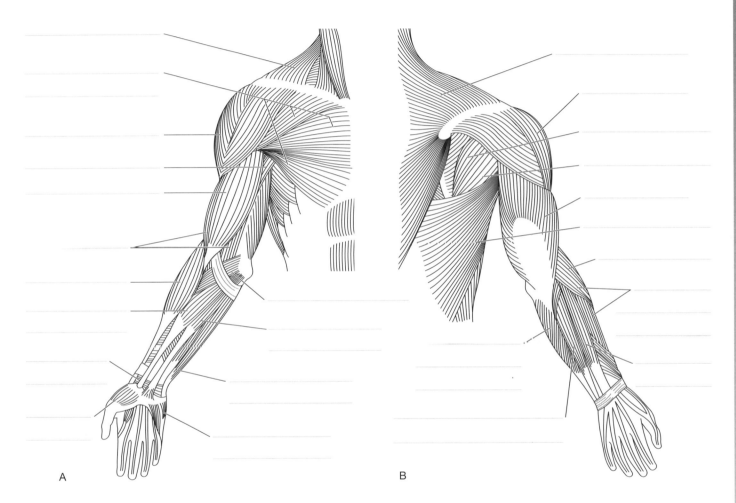

Figure 16.25 The main muscles that move the joints of the upper limb. A. Anterior view. B. Posterior view

MUSCLES OF THE LOWER LIMBS

  Colouring and labelling

80. Colour and label the muscles of the lower limb shown in Figure 16.26.

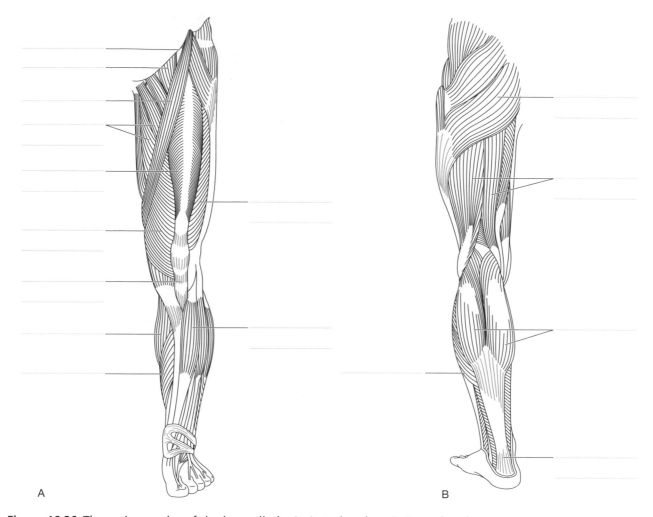

A   B

Figure 16.26 The main muscles of the lower limb. A. Anterior view. B. Posterior view

MUSCLES OF THE PELVIC FLOOR

  Colouring and matching

81. Colour and match the following parts of the pelvic floor on Figure 16.27:

○ External anal sphincter

○ Coccygeus

○ Levator ani

○ Coccyx

○ Vaginal orifice

○ Anal orifice

○ Urethral orifice

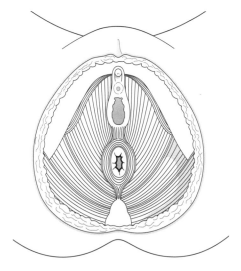

Figure 16.27 The muscles of the female pelvic floor

82. Outline the function of the pelvic floor.

_____

_____

_____.

17 Introduction to genetics

Genetics is the study of genes, which direct the function of body cells, and transmit hereditary information from one generation to the next (heredity).

? MCQs

1. A diploid cell has: ___C___.

   a. 23 chromosomes
   b. no nucleus
   c. 22 pairs of autosomes
   d. two X-chromosomes.

2. Which of the following describes the structural hierarchy of the genetic material of the cell, starting with the largest? _____.

   a. DNA, gene, nucleotide, chromosome
   b. Gene, chromosome, DNA, nucleotide
   c. Chromosome, gene, DNA, nucleotide
   d. Nucleotide, DNA, chromosome, gene.

3. Of the X and Y chromosomes, which of the following is NOT true? ___d___.

   a. these are the sex chromosomes
   b. in the cell karyotype, they are pair number 23
   c. gametes carry one or the other
   d. they carry no genes of significance.

4. Genes: ___a___.

   a. normally exist in pairs, called alleles
   b. are not found in red blood cells or skeletal muscle   cells
   c. carry information that codes for carbohydrate production
   d. always exist in the same form at each locus.

? Pot luck

5. What do the following terms stand for?

   a. DNA- _____

   b. RNA- _____

✎ Completion

6. The paragraph below describes the structure and function of DNA. Complete the paragraph by filling in the blanks.

The nucleus contains the body's _____ material, in the form of DNA, which is built from nucleotides, each made up of three components: a _____ group, the sugar _____ and one of four _____. DNA is a double strand of nucleotides that resembles a _____, or twisted ladder. DNA and associated proteins, also called _____, are coiled together, forming _____. During cell division, the DNA becomes very tightly coiled and can be seen as _____ under the microscope. There are _____ pairs of them in most human cells. Each consists of many functional subunits called _____. Any given type of cell uses only part of the whole genetic code, also called the _____, to carry out its specific activities. Each _____ contains the genetic code, or instructions, for the synthesis of one _____, that could, for example, be an _____ needed to catalyse a particular chemical _____, a hormone, or it may form part of the structure of a cell. The coded instructions have to be transferred to the _____ of the cell, since that is where the organelles that make protein, the _____, are found. DNA itself does not transfer, but a copy of the genetic code is made in the form of _____, which leaves the _____. When its instructions have been read and the new protein synthezised, the copy is destroyed.

Matching, colouring and completion

7. Figure 17.1 shows a section of DNA. Colour the sugar and phosphate groups in the backbone different colours.

8. Complete the base sequence on strand 1 in Fig. 17.1 by drawing in and colouring the bases to complement strand 2.

9. For the following base sequence in a single strand of DNA, work out the corresponding sequence:

   a. in the other strand of the DNA molecule, and
   b. of a piece of mRNA made from this DNA.

   Use this information to complete Table 17.1.

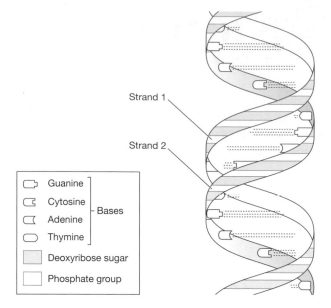

Figure 17.1 Deoxyribonucleic acid (DNA)

DNA Strand 1	C	C	G	T	A	A	C	T	C	A	A	T	G	T
DNA Strand 2														
mRNA														

Table 17.1 The DNA code

 Labelling

10. Figure 17.2 shows the mechanism of protein synthesis from the DNA code. Label the structures indicated.

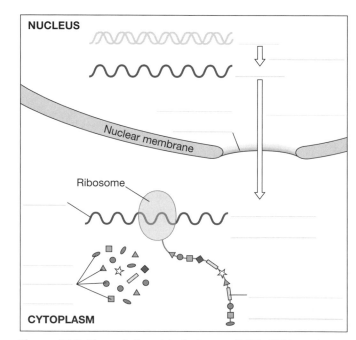

Figure 17.2 The relationship between DNA, RNA and protein synthesis

Matching

11. The list below describes characteristics of the nucleic acids. Decide whether each characteristic applies to DNA, RNA or both by writing DNA, RNA or Both against each item.

a. Contains uracil _____

b. Contains deoxyribose sugar _____

c. Contains phosphate _____

d. Its information is read by translation _____

e. Contains thymine _____

f. Contains ribose sugar _____

g. Is destroyed after its message is read _____

h. Is single stranded _____

i. Contains guanine _____

j. Its information is read by transcription _____

? **Pot luck**

12. Of the following eight statements, only four are correct. Identify the incorrect statements and write the corrected version in the spaces provided.

a. Translation takes place in the nucleus.

b. The base code in DNA is read in triplets.

c. A codon is a piece of DNA carrying information.

d. Stop and start codons initiate and terminate protein synthesis.

e. All new proteins made by a cell must be used within that cell.

f. All body cells contain an identical copy of the genome.

g. In each cell, genes whose function is not required are kept switched off.

h. Proteins are built on ribosomes in the cytoplasm.

_____

_____

_____

_____

_____

_____

_____

_____

 Completion

13. Table 17.2 relates to mitosis and meiosis. Complete it by filling in the appropriate boxes.

Table 17.2 Characteristics of mitosis and meiosis

	Mitosis	Meiosis
One division or two?	One	two
Daughter cells diploid or haploid?	Diploid	haploid
Does crossing over take place?	No	Yes
Are daughter cells identical to parent?	Yes	No
Two or four cells produced?	Two	Four
Are daughter cells identical to one another?	Yes	No
Which process produces gametes?		Meiosis
Which process replaces damaged cells?	Mitosis	

14. The following paragraph relates to autosomal inheritance. Complete it by scoring out the incorrect options in bold.

    One chromosome of each pair is inherited from the mother and one from the father, so there are **two/~~four~~** copies of each gene in the cell. Two chromosomes of the same pair are called ~~homologues~~/**homozygotes/autosomes**, and the genes are present in paired sites called **chromatids/~~traits~~/~~alleles~~**.
    When the paired genes are identical, they are called **homozygous/~~heterozygous~~**, but if they are different forms they are called **~~homozygous~~/heterozygous**. Dominant genes are always ~~present on the maternal chromosome~~/**expressed over recessive genes**/~~found in pairs~~. Individuals homozygous for a dominant gene **can/~~cannot~~** pass the recessive form on to their children, and individuals heterozygous for a gene **can/~~cannot~~** pass on either form of the gene to theirs.

 Definitions

Define the following terms:

15. Phenotype _____

    _____

16. Genotype _____

    _____

 Completion

17. Complete the Punnett square (Box 17.1) to illustrate the possible combinations of genes in the children of parents both heterozygous for the ability to roll their tongue. Use T=dominant gene; t=recessive gene.

Box 17.1

Father's genes

Mother's genes

18. Which of the genotypes above will give a tongue-rolling child? _____

19. Which of the genotypes in Box 17.1 are homozygous? _____

20. Complete the Punnett square (Box 17.2) to illustrate the possible combinations of genes in the children of a mother homozygous for the recessive gene for blue eyes, and a father homozygous for the dominant gene for brown eyes. Use B=brown eyes, b=blue eyes.

Box 17.2

Father's genes

Mother's genes

21. If the parents have four children, one each of the genotypes above, how many blue-eyed children will they have? _____

22. Red-green colour blindness is inherited on the X-chromosome (sex-linkage). Complete the Punnett square (Box 17.3), to show the possible combinations of genes in the children of a colour-blind mother and a normally sighted father. Don't forget to include the sex chromosomes (XX and XY); use B=normal gene, b=colour-blind gene as superscripts, e.g. X^B.

Box 17.3

Father's genes

Mother's genes

23. What is the male:female ratio in the children above? _____.

24. What percentage of the boys will be colour blind?

    _____

25. What term is used to describe the genetic condition of the girls? _____

18 The reproductive system

The reproductive systems in men and women are built differently, although their common function is primarily to ensure production of children and the passing on of the parents' genetic material into another generation. Both systems produce gametes, or sex cells, which fuse to form a potential human being. Females have the additional role of protecting the developing baby within the womb, giving birth and nourishing it in the months after birth. This chapter will test your understanding of the structures and processes involved.

THE FEMALE REPRODUCTIVE SYSTEM

 Labelling

1. Figure 18.1 shows the female external genitalia. Label the structures shown.

2. Indicate the position of the perineal area on Figure 18.1

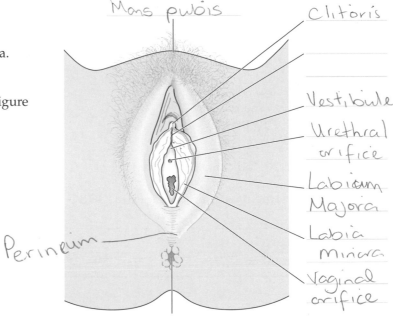

Figure 18.1 Female external genitalia

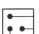 **Labelling, colouring and matching**

3. Figure 18.2 shows the internal female reproductive organs. Label the structures indicated.

4. On Figure 18.2, colour and match the following:

○ Uterus
○ Uterine tubes
○ Ovary
○ Vagina
○ Broad ligament

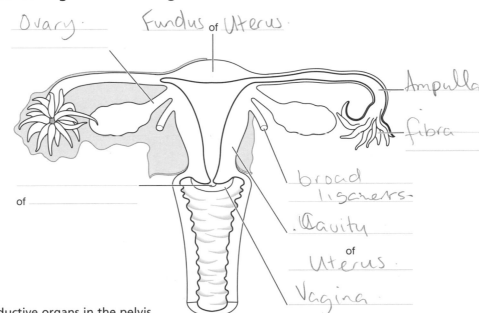

Figure 18.2 The female reproductive organs in the pelvis

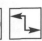 **Labelling, colouring and matching**

5. Figure 18.3 shows the female reproductive organs and some associated structures in the pelvis. Colour and match the following structures:

○ Bladder
○ Peritoneum
○ Pubic bone
○ Sigmoid colon and rectum
○ Vertebrae

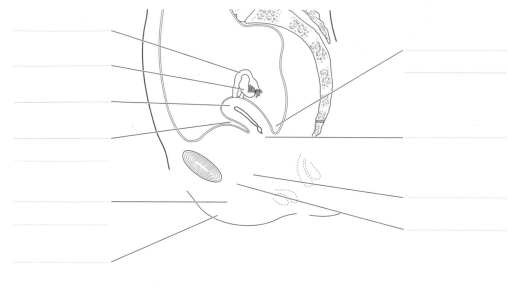

Figure 18.3 Lateral view of the female reproductive organs in the pelvis

6. Label the structures indicated on Figure 18.3.

7. In which of the structures indicated on Figure 18.3 is the pH kept between 4.9 and 3.5, and why?

_____

_____

_____

  Labelling, colouring and matching

8. Figure 18.4 shows a section through the uterus. Colour and match the three layers of the uterine wall:

○ Endometrium
○ Myometrium
○ Perimetrium

9. Label the structures shown on Figure 18.4.

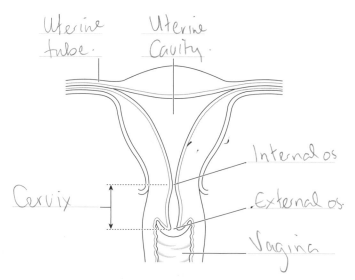

Figure 18.4 A section through the uterus

MCQs

10. Which tissue forms the perimetrium? __b__.

    a. Smooth muscle   **b.** Peritoneum   **c.** Adipose   **d.** Endometrium.

11. Which of the following represents a function of the uterus (choose all that apply)? __a,b,c__.

    a. Nourishment of the ovum   **c.** Expulsion of the baby at term
    b. Production of pregnancy-related hormones   **d.** Attachment of the placenta.

12. What type of tissue lines the uterine tubes? __c,d__.

    a. Delicate areolar to protect the ovum   **c.** Fimbriae, to waft the ovum towards the uterus
    b. Smooth muscle, which contracts rhythmically   **d.** Ciliated epithelium, for propulsion of the ovum.
        to push the ovum along

13. Which of the following is true concerning the uterine tubes? __d__.

    a. They are covered by the round ligament   **c.** They are supplied with blood by the pudendal arteries
    b. They make direct contact with the ovaries   **d.** Fertilization normally takes place here.
        at their lateral ends

   Labelling, colouring and matching

14. Figure 18.5 shows the main stages of development of a single ovarian follicle. Colour, match and label the following structures as you follow through the process:

    ○ Primordial follicle
    ○ Follicle approaching maturity
    ○ Mature ovarian follicle
    ○ Ovum within follicle
    ○ Corpus luteum forming
    ○ Fully formed corpus luteum
    ○ Fibrous corpus albicans

15. On Figure 18.5, indicate the times within an average ovarian cycle that each of these stages would be reached by completing the time scale in the open ovals around the ovary.

16. Name the process taking place at A.

    __Ovulation__

17. Complete Figure 18.5 by labelling the remaining structures indicated.

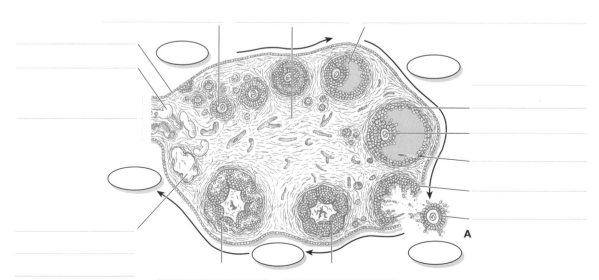

Figure 18.5 Stages of follicular development within the ovary

Completion

18. The following paragraph describes the control of ovarian function. Score out the incorrect options in bold, leaving the correct one.

Maturation of the follicle is stimulated by ~~luteinizing hormone~~/follicle stimulating hormone/ ~~progesterone~~ released by the anterior pituitary, and oestrogen from the **follicular cells**/~~anterior pituitary~~/~~placenta~~. Ovulation is triggered by a surge of ~~luteinizing hormone releasing hormone~~/luteinizing hormone/~~oestrogen~~, which is secreted by the anterior pituitary. This release takes place a few **minutes**/**hours**/**days** before ovulation. After ovulation, the now empty follicle develops into the ~~primordial follicle~~/~~corpus albicans~~/corpus luteum, and its main function is to secrete ~~progesterone~~/~~oestrogen~~/progesterone and oestrogen, which maintain(s) the uterine lining in case fertilization and implantation occur. If pregnancy does occur, the embedded ovum supports the corpus luteum by producing **human chorionic gonadotrophin**/~~luteinzing hormone~~/~~oestrogen~~, which keeps it functioning for the next 3 months or so, until the ~~corpus albicans~~/placenta/~~umbilical cord~~ is developed enough to take on this role. If pregnancy does not occur, the corpus luteum degenerates and forms a scar on the surface of the ovary called the ~~liquor folliculi~~/corpus albicans/~~germinal epithelium~~.

 Pot luck

19. List the main changes that take place in the female body during puberty:

- Breast tissue develops.
- Menstruation begins.
- Pubic hair grows.
- Skin becomes greasy - Spots/acne
- _____
- _____

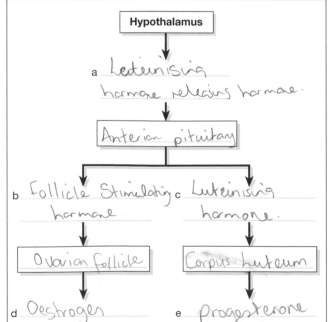

 Completion

20. Figure 18.6 summarizes the main female reproductive hormones and the glands that synthesize them. Complete the figure by filling in the names of the glands (in the boxes) and the hormones a, b, c, d and e.

21. For each of the hormones named in question 19, describe their main functions:

a. _____
_____
_____

b. _____
_____
_____

c. _____
_____
_____

d. _____
_____
_____

e. _____
_____
_____

Figure 18.6 Female reproductive hormones and target tissues

Labelling, colouring and matching

35. Figure 18.10 shows sections through the testis. Figure 18.10A shows the coverings of the testis, and 18.10B shows the relationship between the testis and the deferent duct (vas deferens). In Figure 18.10A, colour and match the different layers around the testis using the key below:

○ Skin
○ Smooth muscle
○ Tunica vaginalis
○ Tunica albuginea
○ Connective tissue forming septum

36. In Figure 18.10B, colour, match and label the following sections of tubule:

○ Convoluted seminiferous tubules
○ Straight seminiferous tubules
○ Efferent ductules

37. Colour and label the remaining structures indicated on Figure 18.10A and B.

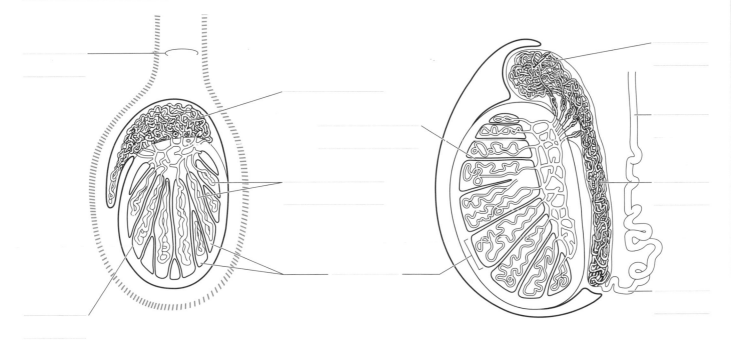

A

B

Figure 18.10 The testis. A. A section through the testis and its coverings; B. A longitudinal section through a testis and its deferent duct

? MCQs

38. How many lobules are found in each testis? _____.

    a. 20–30   **b.** 100–150   **c.** 200–300   **d.** 1000–2000.

39. What is the function of the interstitial cells (of Leydig)? _____.

    a. Production of sperm
    b. Manufacture of nutrients for sperm
    c. Supporting connective cells
    d. Synthesis of testosterone.

40. Sperm are produced from the: _____.

    a. Intersitial cells between the seminiferous tubules
    b. Germinal epithelium of the seminiferous tubules
    c. Head of the epididymis
    d. Spermatic cord.

41. Which of the following is true of spermatozoa? _____.

    a. Sperm production is most efficient at temperatures greater than body temperature

    b. The body of the spermatozoon contains mainly DNA

    c. The head of the spermatozoon is rich in mitochondria, to provide energy for the tail

    d. The hormone promoting sperm production is FSH, from the anterior pituitary.

42. Which of the following is not found within the spermatic cord? _____.

    a. Testicular artery   **b.** Germinal epithelium   **c.** Deferent duct   **d.** Smooth muscle.

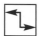 ## Colouring and matching

43. Figure 18.11 shows a section through the prostate gland and some associated structures. Colour and match the following:

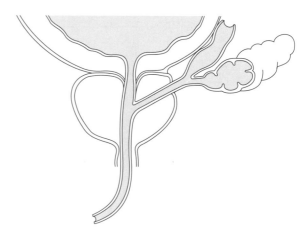

○ Wall of the urinary bladder
○ Ejaculatory duct
○ Urethra
○ Deferent duct
○ Seminal vesicle
○ Prostate gland

Figure 18.11 Section through the prostate gland and associated structures

 ## Completion

44. Complete Table 18.2.

	% sperm volume	Function
Spermatozoa		
Prostate secretions		
Seminal vesicle secretions		

Table 18.2 Nature and function of sperm volume

1 The body as a whole

ANSWERS

1. The study of body structure and the physical relationships between body parts.

2. The study of how the body parts work and the ways they cooperate to maintain life and health.

3. The study of abnormalities and how they affect body function.

4.

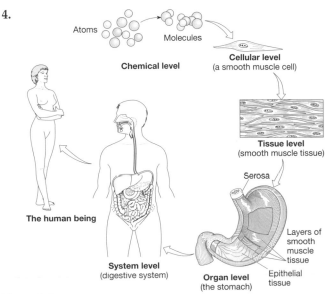

Figure 1.1

5. Table 1.1 Levels of structural complexity and their characteristics

Level of structural complexity	Characteristics
The human being	Comprises many systems that work interdependently to maintain health
Organ level	Carries out a specific function and is composed of different types of tissue
Cellular level	The smallest independent units of living matter
System level	Consists of one or more organs and contributes to one or more survival needs of the body
Chemical level	Atoms and molecules that form the building blocks of larger substances
Tissue level	A group of cells with similar structures and functions

6. The **external** environment surrounds the body and provides the oxygen and nutrients required by all body cells. The **skin** provides a barrier between the **dry** external environment and the **watery** internal environment. The **internal** environment is the medium in which the body cells exist. Cells are bathed in fluid called **interstitial** fluid, also known as **tissue** fluid. The **cell membrane** provides a potential barrier to substances entering or leaving cells. This prevents **large** molecules moving between the cell and interstitial fluid. **Small** particles can usually pass through the membrane more easily and therefore the chemical composition of the fluid inside the cell is different from that outside.

7.

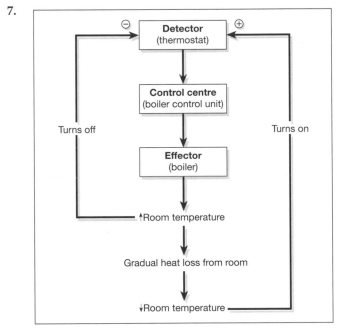

Figure 1.2

8. The composition of the internal environment is maintained within narrow limits, and this fairly constant state is called **homeostasis**. In systems controlled by negative feedback mechanisms, the effector response **reverses** the effect of the original stimulus. When body temperature falls below the preset level, specialized temperature-sensitive nerve endings act as **detectors** and relay this information to cells in the hypothalamus of the brain that form the **control centre**. This results in activation of **effector** responses that raise body temperature. When body temperature returns to the **normal** range again, the temperature-sensitive nerve endings no longer stimulate the cells in the hypothalamus and the heat conserving mechanisms are switched off.

9. Shivering; narrowing of the blood vessels supplying the skin (vasoconstriction); behavioural changes, e.g. putting on more clothes, moving nearer a source of heat.

10. Water and electrolyte concentrations, pH of body fluids, blood glucose levels, blood pressure, blood and tissue oxygen and carbon dioxide levels.

11. It is an amplifier or cascade system where the stimulus progressively increases the response until stimulation ceases.

12. a. Respiratory. b. Digestive. c. Skin (integumentary system).

13. a. Digestive. b. Urinary. c. Respiratory.

14. Non-specific defence mechanisms provide protection against a wide range of invaders, e.g. the skin, mucus from mucous membranes and gastric juice, whereas specific defence mechanisms afford protection against one particular invader (an antigen) and response is through the immune system.

15. a. F, b. T, c. T.

16. The childbearing years begin at **puberty** and end at the **menopause**. During this time an **ovum** matures in the ovary about every **28** days. If **fertilization** takes place the zygote embeds itself in the **uterus** and grows to maturity during pregnancy, or **gestation**, in about **40** weeks. If fertilization does not occur it passes out of the body accompanied by bleeding, called **menstruation**.

17. Carrying to or towards the centre, e.g. central nervous system.

18. Carrying away or away from the centre, e.g. central nervous system.

19. A substance that is recognized as foreign by the immune system, e.g. animal hair, pollen, microorganisms.

20. An abnormally powerful response to an antigen that usually poses no threat to the body.

21.

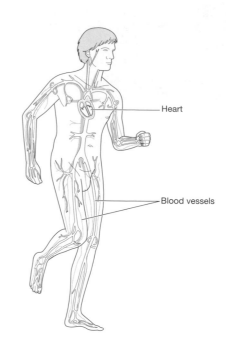

Figure 1.3

22. and 23.

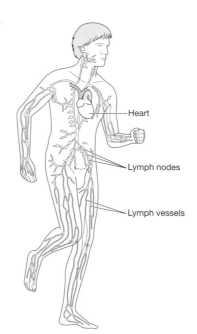

Figure 1.4

24. and 25.

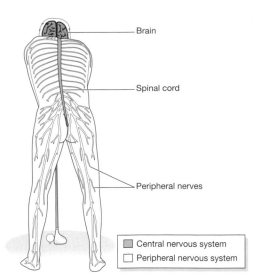

Figure 1.5

28.

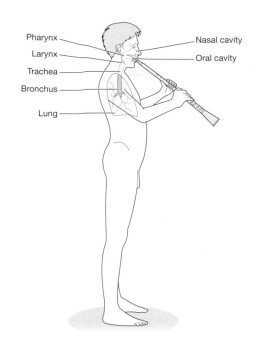

Figure 1.6

26. The endocrine system consists of a number of **glands** in various parts of the body. The glands synthesize and secrete chemical messengers called **hormones** into the **bloodstream**. These chemicals stimulate **target organs/tissues**. Changes in hormone levels are usually controlled by **negative feedback** mechanisms. The endocrine system, in conjunction with part of the **nervous** system, controls **involuntary** body function. Changes involving the latter system are usually **fast** while those of the endocrine system tend to be **slow** and precise.

27. Table 1.2 The special senses and their related sensory organs

Special sense	Related sensory organ
Sight	Eye
Hearing	Ear
Balance	Ear
Smell	Nose
Taste	Tongue

29.

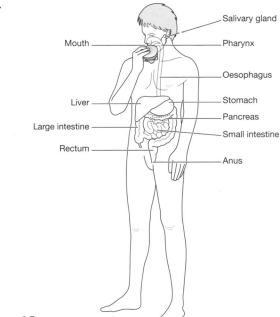

Figure 1.7

30.

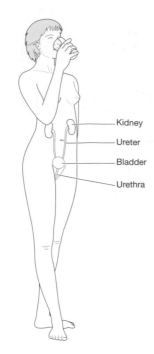

Figure 1.8

31.

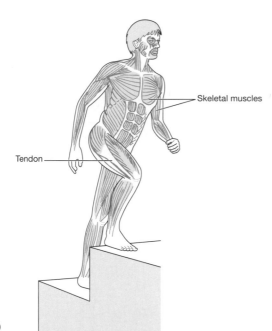

Figure 1.9

32.

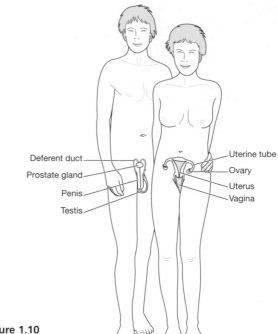

Figure 1.10

33. Building up or synthesis of large and complex chemical substances.

34. Breaking down of large chemical substances.

35. Elimination of urine, voiding.

36. Elimination of faeces.

37. a. Symptom. b. Congenital. c. Acquired. d. Chronic. e. Syndrome. f. Acute. g. Sign.

38. The cause of disease.

39. The nature of a disease and its effect on body functioning.

40. The likely outcome of a disease.

41. A disease or condition of which the cause is unknown.

2 Electrolytes and body fluids

ANSWERS

1. The smallest particle of an element that exists in a stable form.

2. A substance containing one or more elements.

3. A chemical containing only one type of atom.

4. and **5.**

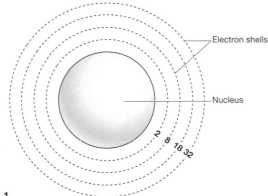

Figure 2.1

6. Table 2.1 Characteristics of subatomic particles

Particle	Mass	Electric charge	Location in atom
Proton	1 unit	1 positive	Within nucleus
Neutron	1 unit	Neutral	Within nucleus
Electron	Negligible	1 negative	Orbiting nucleus

7. 2.8.18., because its outer shell contains the maximum number of electrons for that shell, conferring stability on the whole atom.

8. The number of protons in the nucleus of the atom.

9. The total number of protons and neutrons in the nucleus of the atom.

10.

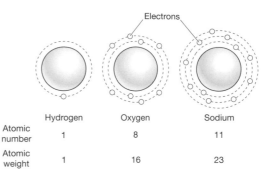

	Hydrogen	Oxygen	Sodium
Atomic number	1	8	11
Atomic weight	1	16	23

Figure 2.2

11. c.

12. b.

13. Table 2.2 Chemical bonds

	Ionic bonds	Covalent bonds
Gives rise to charged particles (ions)	✓	
Commonest bond		✓
Atoms transfer their electrons	✓	
Links sodium and chloride in a molecule of sodium chloride	✓	
Stable bond		✓
Atoms share their electrons		✓
There is no change in the number of protons or neutrons	✓	✓
The weaker of the two bonds	✓	
Links hydrogen and oxygen in a water molecule		✓

14. Electrolytes conduct electricity, exert osmotic pressure and function in acid–base balance.

15. c.

16. b.

17. d.

18. d.

19. Lungs and kidneys.

20. An excess of hydrogen ions, or an excessive fall in the pH of a body fluid or the tissues.

21. CO_2 (carbon dioxide) + H_2O (water)$\leftrightarrow H_2CO_3$ (carbonic acid)$\leftrightarrow H^+$ (hydrogen ion) + HCO_3^- (bicarbonate ion).

22. Table 2.3 Characteristics of some important biological molecules

23.

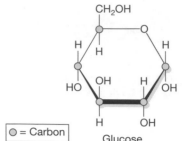

Figure 2.3   ◎ = Carbon   Glucose

24. Source of energy for immediate use by cells; energy storage for body; used to build nucleic acids; act as cell surface receptors.

25.

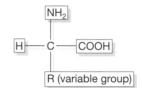

Figure 2.4

	Carbohydrates	Proteins	Nucleotides	Lipids
Building blocks are amino acids		✓		
Contain carbon	✓	✓	✓	✓
Molecules joined with glycosidic linkages	✓			
Used to build genetic material	✓		✓	
Building blocks are monosaccharides	✓			
Contain glycerol				✓
Contain hydrogen	✓	✓	✓	✓
Molecules joined together with peptide bonds		✓		
Strongly hydrophobic				✓
Built from sugar unit, phosphate group and base			✓	
Enzymes are made from these		✓		
Contain oxygen	✓	✓	✓	✓

26. Insulin; haemoglobin; antibodies; enzymes; collagen.

27.

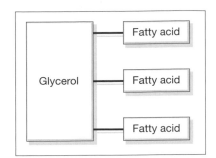

Figure 2.5

28. a. The **fats are a type of lipid** and include certain vitamins (e.g. vitamin A) and hormones (e.g. steroids).
b. and c. are true.
d. Lipid molecules are strongly **hydrophobic**, meaning water hating, leading to an inability to dissolve in water.

29.

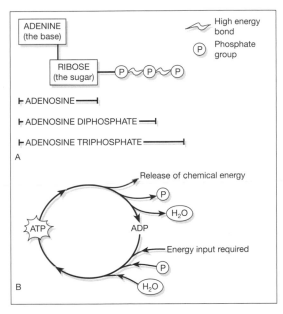

Figure 2.6

30. Enzymes are **proteins** that are used in the body to **speed up** the rates of chemical reactions on which the body's metabolism depends. They are **not** themselves normally used up in the reactions they participate in and are usually fairly specific in the reactions they control. They can either cause two or more molecules to bind together (a **synthetic** reaction) or cause the breaking up of a molecule into smaller groups (a **catabolic** or **breakdown** reaction). The molecule(s) entering the reaction are called **reactants** and they bind to a reactive site on the enzyme molecule called the **active** site. They are bound for only a fraction of a second, but when they are released the reaction has occurred and the new forms of the reactants are now called **products**.

31. b.

32. a.

33. d.

34. a., b., d.

35. 60%.

36. Cytoplasm, potassium, ATP.

3 The cells, tissues, organization of the body

ANSWERS

1. and 2.

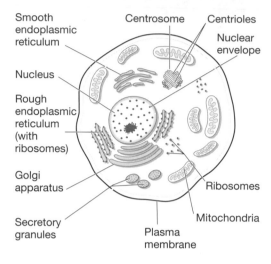

Smooth endoplasmic reticulum
Centrosome
Centrioles
Nuclear envelope
Nucleus
Rough endoplasmic reticulum (with ribosomes)
Golgi apparatus
Secretory granules
Plasma membrane
Ribosomes
Mitochondria

Figure 3.1

3. Table 3.1 Intracellular organelles and their functions

Organelle	Function
Nucleus	The largest organelle, directs the activities of the cell
Mitochondria	Sausage-shaped structures often described as the powerhouse of the cell. Sites of aerobic respiration
Ribosomes	Tiny granules consisting of RNA and protein that synthesize proteins for use within cells
Rough endoplasmic reticulum (ER)	Proteins exported from cells are manufactured here
Smooth endoplasmic reticulum	Lipids and steroid hormones are synthesized here
Golgi apparatus	Stacks of closely flattened membranous sacs that form membrane-bound granules called secretory vesicles
Lysosomes	Secretory granules that contain enzymes for the breakdown of large cellular wastes, e.g. fragments of old organelles
Microfilaments	The tiny strands of protein that provide the structural support and shape of a cell
Microtubules	Contractile proteins involved in movement of cells and of organelles within cells

4. The plasma membrane consists of two layers of phospholipids with some **protein** molecules embedded in them. The phospholipid molecules have a head which is electrically charged and hydrophilic (meaning water **loving**) and a tail that has no charge and is hydrophobic. The phospholipid bilayer is arranged like a sandwich with the hydrophilic heads on the **outside** and the hydrophobic tails on the **inside**. These differences influence the passage of substances across the membrane.

5. Most body cells have one nucleus. Exceptions are mature **red blood** cells (**erythrocytes**), which have none, and **skeletal muscle** cells that may have several. The nucleus is contained within the **nuclear envelope**, a membrane that has **pores**, which allow passage of substances between the nucleus and the **cytoplasm**. It contains the body's **genetic** material, which consists of 46 **chromosomes**, built from **DNA**.

6., 7. and **8.** see Fig. 3.2

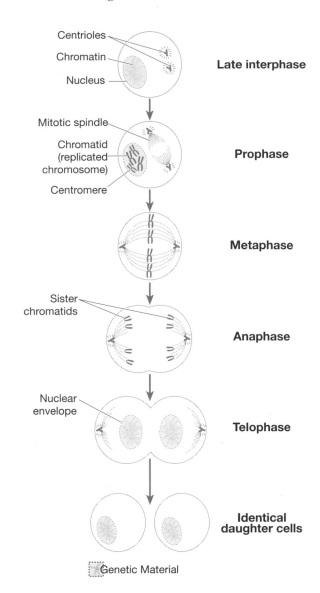

Figure 3.2

9. a. F, **b.** T, **c.** F, **d.** F, **e.** F, **f.** T.

10. Transport up a concentration gradient that requires chemical energy (ATP).

11. Transport down a concentration gradient without the use of chemical energy (ATP).

12. b.   **13.** a.   **14.** d.   **15.** a.   **16.** b.   **17.** c.

18. Transfer of large particles across the plasma membrane into the cell occurs by **phagocytosis** and **pinocytosis**. The particles are engulfed by extensions of the **plasma membrane** that enclose them forming a membrane-bound **vacuole**. Then **lysosomes** adhere to the cell membrane releasing **enzymes** that **digest** the contents. Extrusion of waste materials by the reverse process is called **exocytosis**.

19., 20. and **21.**

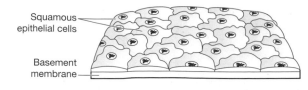

(a)   Squamous epithelium

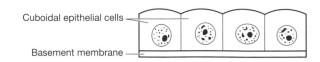

(b)   Cuboidal epithelium

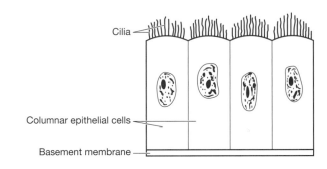

(c)   Ciliated columnar epithelium

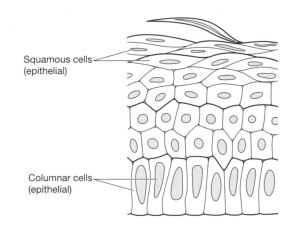

(d)   Stratified epithelium

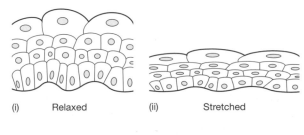

(i)   Relaxed   (ii)   Stretched

(e)   Transitional epithelium

Figure 3.3 (a–e)

22., 23. and 24.

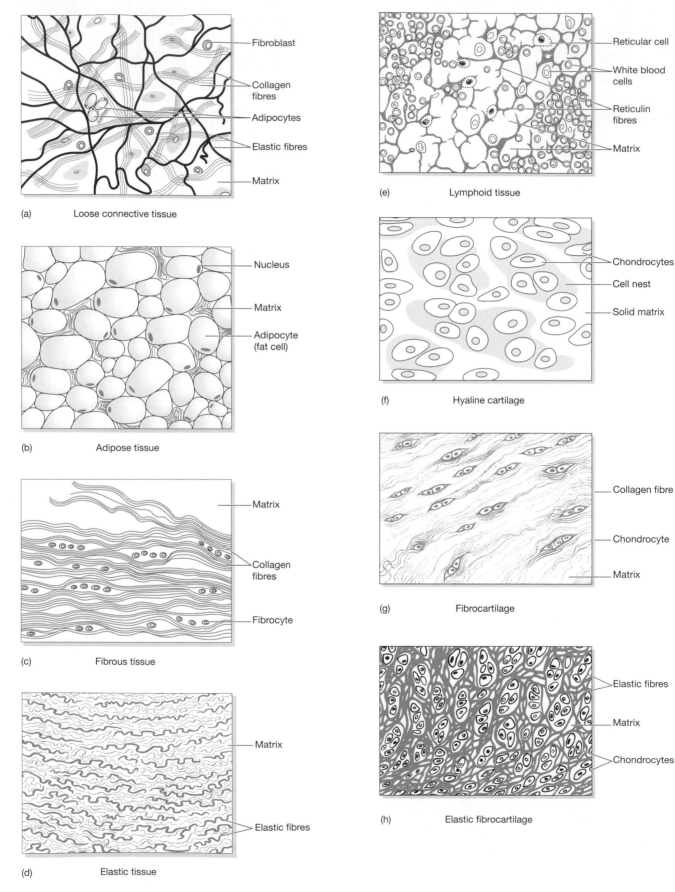

(a) Loose connective tissue

(b) Adipose tissue

(c) Fibrous tissue

(d) Elastic tissue

(e) Lymphoid tissue

(f) Hyaline cartilage

(g) Fibrocartilage

(h) Elastic fibrocartilage

Figure 3.4 (a–h)

25., 26. and **27.** see Figure 3.5

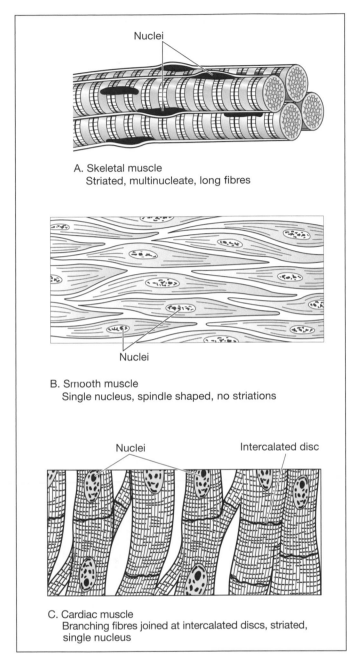

A. Skeletal muscle
Striated, multinucleate, long fibres

Nuclei

B. Smooth muscle
Single nucleus, spindle shaped, no striations

Nuclei   Intercalated disc

C. Cardiac muscle
Branching fibres joined at intercalated discs, striated,
single nucleus

Figure 3.5

28. Muscle cells are also called **fibres**. Muscle tissue has the property of **contractility** that brings about movement, both within the body and of the body itself. This requires a blood supply to provide **oxygen**, **calcium** and **nutrients**, and to remove **wastes**. The chemical energy needed is derived from **ATP**.

Skeletal muscle is also known as **voluntary** muscle because **contraction** is under conscious control. When examined under the microscope, the cells are roughly **cylindrical** in shape and may be as long as **35 cm**. The cells show a pattern of clearly visible stripes, also known as **striations**. Skeletal muscle is stimulated by **motor nerve** impulses that originate in the brain or spinal cord and end at the **neuromuscular junction**.

Smooth muscle has the intrinsic ability to **contract** and **relax**, but it can also be stimulated by **autonomic nerve** impulses, some **hormones** and **local metabolites**.

Cardiac muscle is found only in the wall of the **heart**, which has its own **pacemaker** system, meaning that this tissue contracts in a co-ordinated manner without external stimulation. **Autonomic nerve** impulses and some **hormones** influence activity of this type of muscle.

29. c.

30. a., b., c.

31. a., c.

32. b., c., d.

33. Mucous membrane is sometimes referred to as the **mucosa**. It forms the moist lining of body tracts, e.g. the **alimentary, respiratory** and **genitourinary** tracts. The membrane consists of **epithelial** cells some of which produce a secretion called **mucus**. This sticky substance protects the lining from **injury**. In the alimentary tract it **lubricates** the contents and in the respiratory system it traps **inhaled particles**.

A serous membrane may also be known as the **serosa**. It consists of a double layer of **loose areolar** connective tissue lined by **simple squamous** epithelium. The layer lining the body cavity is the **parietal** layer and that surrounding organs within a cavity, the **visceral** layer. There are three sites where serous membranes are found:

a. the **pleura** lining the thoracic cavity and surrounding the lungs
b. the **pericardium** lining the pericardial cavity and surrounding the heart
c. the **peritoneum** lining the abdominal cavity and surrounding the abdominal organs.

Synovial membrane lines the cavities of **moveable (synovial) joints**. It consists of **areolar connective** tissue containing **elastic** fibres. This membrane secretes a clear, sticky, oily substance known as **synovial fluid**. It provides **lubrication** and **nourishment**, and prevents **friction** between structures in **synovial** joints.

34. and 35.

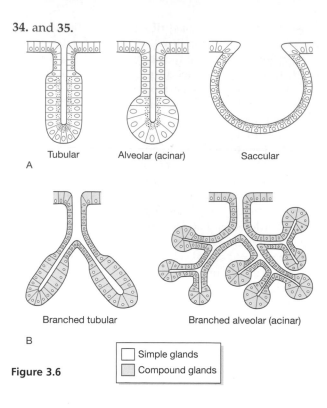

A
Tubular   Alveolar (acinar)   Saccular

B
Branched tubular   Branched alveolar (acinar)

	Simple glands
	Compound glands

Figure 3.6

36. This is the position assumed in all anatomical descriptions to ensure accuracy and consistency. The body is in the **upright** position with the head facing **forwards**, the arms facing **forwards** with the palms of the hands facing **forwards** and the feet **together**.

37. and 38.

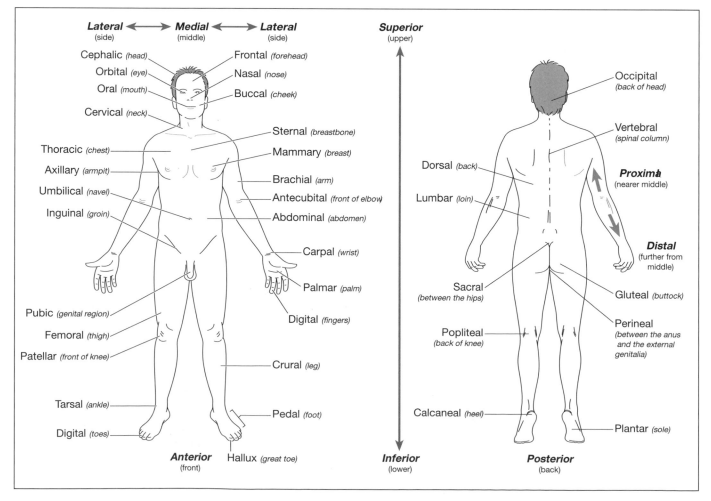

Figure 3.7

39. and 40.

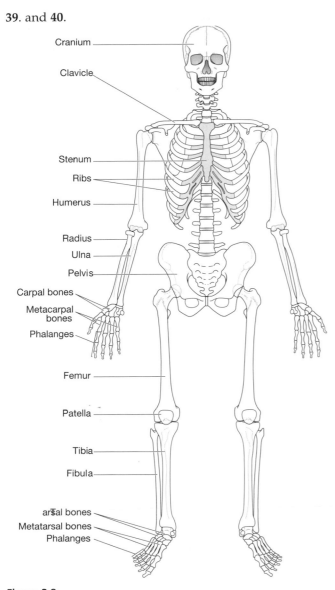

Cranium
Clavicle
Stenum
Ribs
Humerus
Radius
Ulna
Pelvis
Carpal bones
Metacarpal bones
Phalanges
Femur
Patella
Tibia
Fibula
arsal bones
Metatarsal bones
Phalanges

Figure 3.8

41.

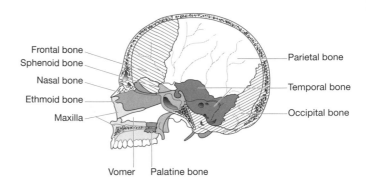

Frontal bone
Sphenoid bone
Nasal bone
Ethmoid bone
Maxilla
Parietal bone
Temporal bone
Occipital bone
Vomer   Palatine bone

Figure 3.9

42.

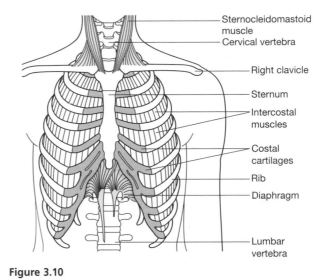

Sternocleidomastoid muscle
Cervical vertebra
Right clavicle
Sternum
Intercostal muscles
Costal cartilages
Rib
Diaphragm
Lumbar vertebra

Figure 3.10

43. and 44.

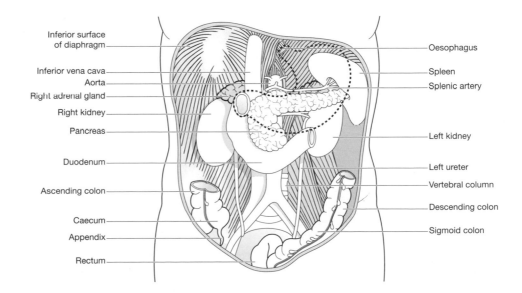

Inferior surface of diaphragm
Inferior vena cava
Aorta
Right adrenal gland
Right kidney
Pancreas
Duodenum
Ascending colon
Caecum
Appendix
Rectum
Oesophagus
Spleen
Splenic artery
Left kidney
Left ureter
Vertebral column
Descending colon
Sigmoid colon

Figure 3.11

45.

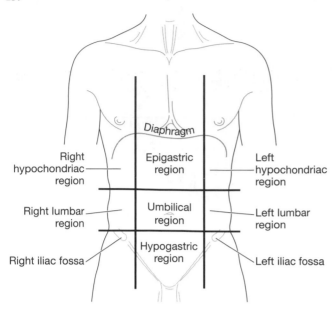

Diaphragm

Right hypochondriac region — — Epigastric region — Left hypochondriac region

Right lumbar region — — Umbilical region — Left lumbar region

Right iliac fossa — Hypogastric region — Left iliac fossa

Figure 3.12

46. a. 5; b. 3; c. 1, 2, 3; d. 1, 2, 3, 4; e. 5; f. 3; g. 1; h. 1; i. 5.

47. a. Abdominal. b. Thoracic. c. Pelvic. d. Abdominal. e. Cranial. f. Pelvic. g. Thoracic. h. Abdominal.

48. An agent that can cause malignant changes in cells.

49. A mass of tissue that has escaped the body's normal growth control mechanisms and usually grows faster than normal.

4 The blood

ANSWERS

1. and **2.**

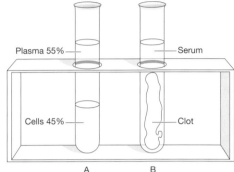

Figure 4.1

3. Clotting proteins.

4. Table 4.1 Components of plasma

These chemicals travel from the gland of origin to distant tissues	Hormones
These provide the building blocks for new tissue proteins	Amino acids
These molecules combat antigens	Antibodies
90–92% of plasma is this	Water
This substance is needed for haemoglobin synthesis	Iron
An important respiratory waste is carried as this	Bicarbonate ion
This participates in the clotting reaction	Fibrinogen
This is needed for healthy bones and teeth	Phosphate
This is the principal fuel source for the tissues	Glucose
This is a nitrogenous waste	Urea

5. b.   **6.** d.   **7.** d.   **8.** b.   **9.** a., d.   **10.** c.

11. and **12.**

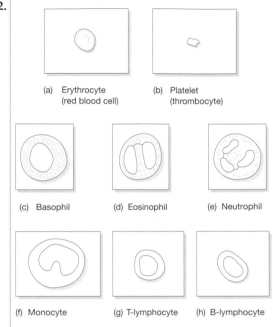

Figure 4.2

13. Haemopoiesis.

14. To make more space for haemoglobin.

15. Enzymes and toxic chemicals (neutrophils and eosinophils); histamine and heparin (basophils).

16. a: 11, 12, 13, 17, 18, 19, 20; **b:** 3, 8, 12, 17, 18; **c:** 1, 4, 17, 18; **d:** 4, 7, 14, 17, 18; **e:** 4, 6, 17, 18; **f:** 5, 9, 16, 17, 18; **g:** 5, 9, 10, 15, 17, 18; **h:** 2, 5, 9, 10, 15, 17, 18.

17. b.   **18.** d.   **19.** a.   **20.** d.   **21.** d.   **22.** b

23.

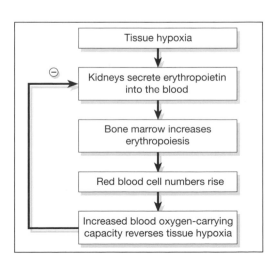

Figure 4.3

24. The life span of red blood cells is usually about **120** days. Their breakdown, also called **haemolysis**, is carried out by phagocytic **reticuloendothelial** cells found mainly in the **liver**, **spleen** and **bone marrow**. Their breakdown releases the mineral **iron**, which is kept by the body and stored in the **liver**. It is used to form new **haemoglobin**. The protein released is converted to the intermediate **biliverdin**, and then to the yellow pigment **bilirubin**, before being bound to plasma protein and transported to the **liver**, where it is excreted in the **bile**.

25. See Table 4.2 The ABO system of blood grouping.

26. O.   27. AB.

28. See Table 4.3 Characteristics of white blood cells.

29. **a.** When platelets come into contact with a damaged vessel wall, they stick to it and release serotonin, which constricts the vessel, slowing blood flow; other agents that constrict the vessel, e.g. thromboxanes, are released by the damaged tissue itself.

b. The sticky platelets clump, releasing agents (e.g. ADP) that bring in more platelets and quickly enlarge the temporary platelet plug.

c. Coagulation (also known as blood clotting) is a complex, multi-stage process involving many different proteins, but the end result is formation of an insoluble mesh of fibrin strands in and around the damaged area of blood vessel wall, which traps red blood cells and forms a strong 'bandage' across the breach.

d. To repair the blood vessel wall, the clot has to be removed; plasminogen is an inactive precursor of the clot-dissolving enzyme plasmin, and is activated to plasmin by plasminogen activator. Gradual removal of the clot is accompanied by healing of the damaged tissues, including the blood vessel wall.

Blood group	Type of antigen present on red cell surface	Type of antibody present in plasma	Can safely donate to:	Can safely receive from:
A	A	Anti-B	A, AB	A, O
B	B	Anti-A	B, AB	B, O
AB	A, B	Neither	AB	AB, A, B, O
O	Neither	A, B	O, A, B, AB	O

Table 4.2 The ABO system of blood grouping

	Neutrophils	Eosinophils	Basophils	Monocytes	Lymphocytes
Phagocyte	✓	✓			
Involved in allergy		✓	✓		
Converted to macrophages				✓	
Release histamine			✓		
Many in lymph nodes					✓
Kupffer cells				✓	
Increased numbers in infections	✓	✓	✓	✓	✓
Kill parasites		✓			
Part of the reticuloendothelial system				✓	

Table 4.3 Characteristics of white blood cells

5 The cardiovascular system

ANSWERS

1. The heart pumps blood into two separate circulatory systems, the **pulmonary** circulation and the **systemic** circulation. The **right** side of the heart pumps blood to the lungs, whereas the **left** side of the heart supplies the rest of the body. The **capillaries** are the sites of exchange of nutrients, gases and wastes. Tissue wastes, including carbon dioxide, pass into the **bloodstream** and the tissues are supplied with **oxygen** and **nutrients**.

2.

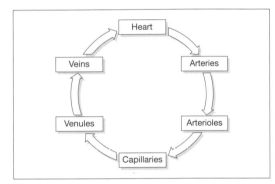

Figure 5.1

3.

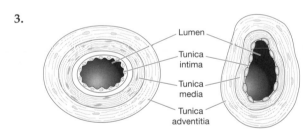

Figure 5.2

4. Table 5.1 Layers of vessel wall

Descriptive phrase	Layer (tunica) of vessel wall
Squamous epithelium	Inner layer (tunica intima)
Contains mainly fibrous tissue	Outer layer (tunica adventitia)
Endothelial layer	Inner layer (tunica intima)
Consists partly of muscle tissue	Middle layer (tunica media)
The vessel's elastic tissue is here	Middle layer (tunica media)
Outer layer	Tunica adventitia

5. b.   **6.** d.   **7.** a.   **8.** c., d.

9. The tiniest arterioles split up into a large number of tinier vessels called **capillaries**. Across the walls of these vessels, the tissues obtain **oxygen** and **nutrients**, and get rid of their **wastes**. The walls of these vessels are therefore thin, being only **one cell** thick. Substances such as **water** and **glucose** can pass across them, whereas larger constituents of blood such as **blood cells** and **plasma proteins** are retained within the vessel. This vast network of microscopic vessels have a diameter of only about **7 μm**, and link the arterioles to the **venules**. In some parts of the body, such as the liver, the vessels in the tissues are wider than this, and are called **sinusoids**. Blood flow here is **slower** than in other tissues because of the bigger lumen.

10. Vasodilation: a., b., d., f., g., i.
Vasoconstriction: c., e., h., j., k., l.

11. c.   **12.** a.   **13.** d.   **14.** b.

15. Table 5.2 Characteristics of osmosis, diffusion and active transport

	Osmosis	Diffusion	Active transport
Movement only down a concentration gradient	✓	✓	
Movement of water molecules	✓		
Movement across a semipermeable membrane	✓	✓	✓
Movement requires energy			✓
Movement up a concentration gradient possible			✓
Movement does not require energy	✓	✓	
Movement of oxygen		✓	
Movement of carbon dioxide		✓	

16. a. Osmotic pressure; b. blood pressure;
c. hydrostatic (blood) pressure; d. hydrostatic (blood) pressure; e. osmotic pressure.

17.

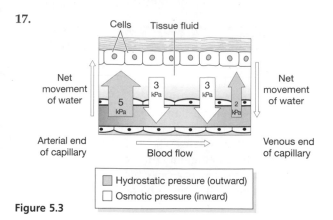

Figure 5.3

18. and 19.

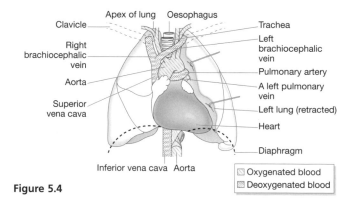

Figure 5.4

20.

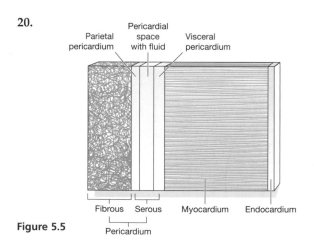

Figure 5.5

21. c.   22. a.   23. d.   24. b.

25. a. Myocardium; b. serous pericardium; c. fibrous pericardium; d. endocardium; e. serous pericardium; f. fibrous pericardium; g. endocardium; h. myocardium; i. serous pericardium; j. myocardium; k. endocardium.

26. Lungs, which are covered with the pleural membrane, and the peritoneal cavity, lined with the peritoneum.

27. and 28.

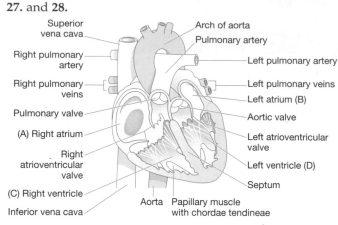

Figure 5.6

29. The chordae tendinae are tendinous cords that fasten the valves to the papillary muscles, and prevent the valves from being pushed into the atria when the ventricles are contracting.

30. The valves prevent backflow of blood in the heart.

31. and 32.

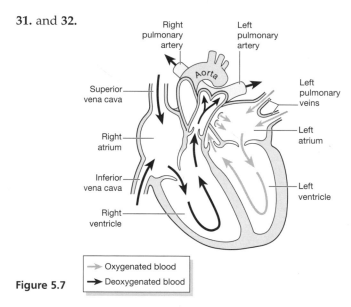

Figure 5.7

33. Aorta, systemic arterial network, capillaries of body tissues, systemic venous network, venae cavae, right atrium, right atrioventricular (tricuspid) valve, right ventricle, pulmonary valve, pulmonary arteries, lungs, pulmonary veins, left atrium, left atrioventricular (mitral) valve, left ventricle, aortic valve, aorta.

34. Because the left ventricle has to pump blood around the systemic circulation, whereas blood from the right is only going as far as the lungs.

35. and 36.

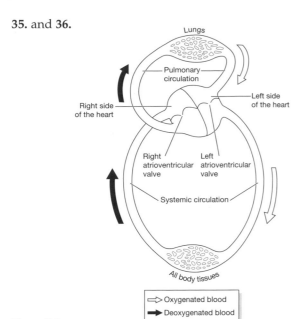

Figure 5.8

37. b. **38.** c. **39.** d. **40.** d.

41.

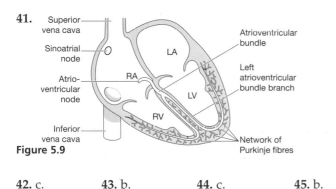

Figure 5.9

42. c. **43.** b. **44.** c. **45.** b.

46. *Diastole*
We will begin this description with the heart in diastole, when the whole heart is **resting**. During this time, in the upper part of the heart, the atria are **relaxed** and blood is flowing **into the atria**. Not only the upper chambers are filling but also the lower ones; because the **atrioventricular** valves are open, we see that the **ventricles** are filling as well. Although blood is travelling into the lower chambers, at this stage the electrical activity has not reached them yet so the ventricles are **relaxed**. Remember, during this period, the heart muscle is not contracting; both the **atria** and the **ventricles** are relaxed.

Atrial systole
The next stage represents atrial systole, or contraction. This is initiated when the **sinoatrial node** fires; its electrical discharge leads to the spread of **electrical impulses** through the atria. Because of the electrical excitation of the muscle, the atria **contract** and this leads to pumping of blood from the **atria** into the **ventricles**. It is important therefore that the

atrioventricular valves are open to permit blood to flow through. The ventricles fill up; because the **aortic** and **pulmonary** valves are closed, blood cannot yet pass from the heart into the great vessels leaving it.

Ventricular systole
The third stage is ventricular systole. The impulse from the sinoatrial node has passed through the atrioventricular node; inspection of the atria shows that they are **relaxed** after their period of activity; this allows them to rest. However, as far as the lower chambers are concerned, because **electrical impulses** are spreading through the **ventricles**, we see that the ventricles **contract**. So that blood cannot flow in a backwards manner into the atria, the **atrioventricular** valves are closed. However, for the ventricles to be able to push blood out of the heart, the **aortic** and **pulmonary** valves **open**. Because of the force generated by the contracting ventricular muscle, blood is pumped from the ventricles into the **pulmonary arteries** and the **aorta**.

The cycle is now complete; the heart will enter another period of diastole, allowing the entire organ to rest briefly before the next period of contraction.

47. b. **48.** a. **49.** d. **50.** c.

51.

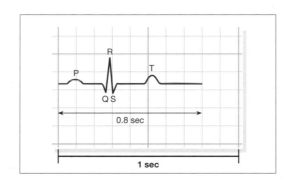

Figure 5.10

52. a. QRS complex; b. P wave; c. T wave; d. QRS complex; e. P wave; f. QRS complex; g. QRS complex; h. QRS complex.

53. 5.6 L. **54.** 80 ml. **55.** 100 beats per minute.

56. a., b., g. **57.** c., d., f., g., h. **58.** c.

59. b. **60.** a. **61.** c.

62. The baroreceptor reflex is important in the **moment-to-moment** control of blood pressure. It is controlled by the cardiovascular centre found in the **medulla oblongata**, and which receives and integrates information from baroreceptors, chemoreceptors and higher centres in the brain. Baroreceptors are receptors sensitive to blood pressure and are found in the **carotid arteries/aorta**. A **rise** in blood pressure activates these receptors, which respond by increasing the activity of **parasympathetic** nerve fibres supplying the heart; this **slows the heart down** and returns the system towards normal. In addition to this, **sympathetic** nerve fibres supplying the blood vessels are **inhibited**, which leads to **vasodilation**, again returning the system towards normal (note that most blood vessels have little or no **parasympathetic** innervation).

On the other hand, if the blood pressure **falls**, baroreceptor activity is decreased, and this also triggers compensatory mechanisms. This time, **sympathetic** activity is increased and this leads to an **increase** in heart rate; in addition, cardiac contractile force is **increased**. The blood vessels respond with **vasoconstriction**; this is mainly due to **increased** activity in **sympathetic** fibres. These measures lead to a restoration of blood pressure towards normal.

In addition to the activity of the baroreceptors described above, chemoreceptors in the **carotid bodies/aorta** measure the pH of the blood. Increase in **carbon dioxide** content of the blood decreases pH and **stimulates** these receptors, leading to an **increase** in stroke volume and heart rate, and a general **vasoconstriction**; this **increases** blood pressure. Other control mechanisms include the renin–angiotensin system, which is involved in **long-term** regulation; activation **increases** blood volume, thereby **increasing** blood pressure.

64. Blood leaving the right ventricle first enters the **pulmonary trunk**, which passes upwards close to the aorta and divides into the right **pulmonary arteries** and the left **pulmonary arteries** at the level of the 5th thoracic vertebra. Each of these branches goes to the corresponding **lung** and enters these organs in the area called the **hilum or root**. Within the tissues, the vessels divide and subdivide, giving a network of many millions of tiny **capillaries**, across the walls of which gases exchange. Blood draining these structures then passes through veins of increasing diameter, which finally unite in the **pulmonary veins**, which carry the blood back to the **left** atrium of the heart.

65.

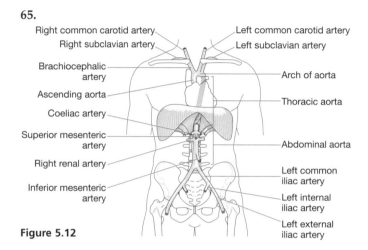

Right common carotid artery
Right subclavian artery
Brachiocephalic artery
Ascending aorta
Coeliac artery
Superior mesenteric artery
Right renal artery
Inferior mesenteric artery

Left common carotid artery
Left subclavian artery
Arch of aorta
Thoracic aorta
Abdominal aorta
Left common iliac artery
Left internal iliac artery
Left external iliac artery

Figure 5.12

66. b.   67. a.   68. b.   69. c.   70. b.   71. c.

72.

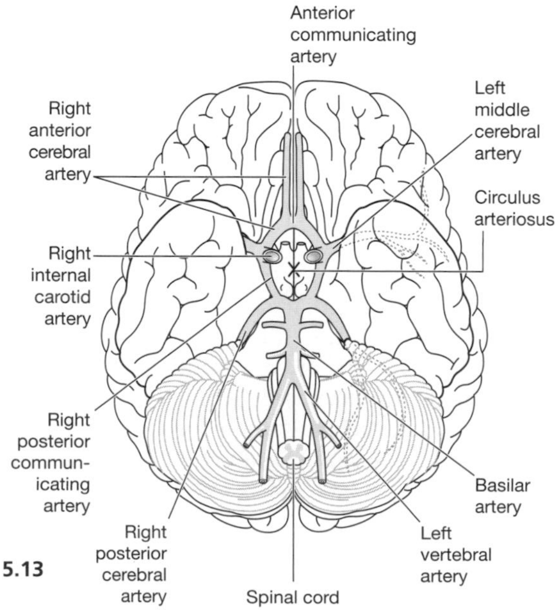

63.

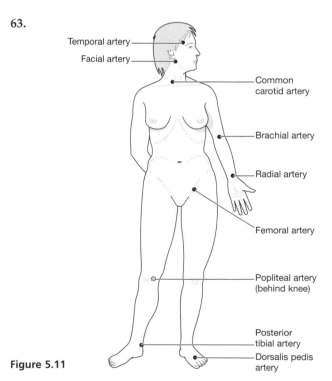

Temporal artery
Facial artery
Common carotid artery
Brachial artery
Radial artery
Femoral artery
Popliteal artery (behind knee)
Posterior tibial artery
Dorsalis pedis artery

Figure 5.11

Anterior communicating artery
Right anterior cerebral artery
Right internal carotid artery
Right posterior communicating artery
Right posterior cerebral artery
Left middle cerebral artery
Circulus arteriosus
Basilar artery
Left vertebral artery
Spinal cord

Figure 5.13

73.

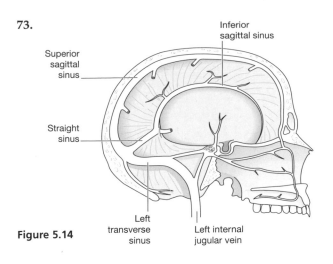

Figure 5.14

75. c.   **76.** d.   **77.** b.   **78.** a.

79. Aorta, common iliac artery, external iliac artery, femoral artery, popliteal artery, anterior tibial artery, dorsalis pedis artery, digital arteries, digital veins, dorsal venous arch, anterior tibial vein, popliteal vein, femoral vein, external iliac vein, common iliac vein, inferior vena cava.

80. d.   **81.** b, c.   **82.** c.   **83.** All of them.   **84.** c.

85. b.   **86.** c.   **87.** b.

74.

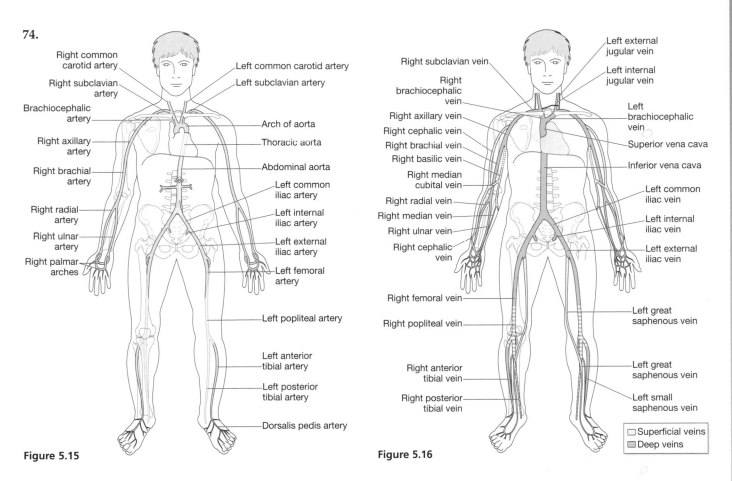

Figure 5.15

Figure 5.16

88 and 89.

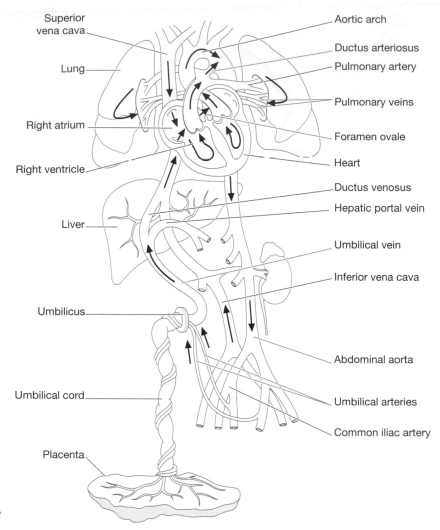

Figure 5.17

90. Produces oestrogen and progesterone to maintain pregnancy; prevents harmful substances crossing into foetal circulation; allows exchange of nutrients and wastes between maternal and foetal circulation.

6 The lymphatic system

ANSWERS

1. and 2.

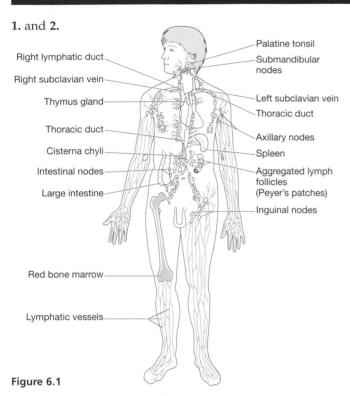

Right lymphatic duct
Right subclavian vein
Thymus gland
Thoracic duct
Cisterna chyli
Intestinal nodes
Large intestine

Palatine tonsil
Submandibular nodes
Left subclavian vein
Thoracic duct
Axillary nodes
Spleen
Aggregated lymph follicles (Peyer's patches)
Inguinal nodes

Red bone marrow

Lymphatic vessels

Figure 6.1

3. a. Tissue drainage; the 3–4 L of fluid that daily escapes from the blood vessels passes into the lymphatic system. b. Absorption of fats into the lacteals of the small intestine. c. Production and maturation of immune cells.

4. b.   **5.** c.   **6.** d.   **7.** c.

8. The smallest lymphatic vessels are called **capillaries**. One significant difference between them and the smallest blood vessels is that they **originate in the tissues**; their function is to drain the lymph, containing **white blood cells**, away from the interstitial spaces. Most tissues have a network of these tiny vessels, but one notable exception is **bone tissue**. The individual tiny vessels join up to form larger ones, which now contain **three** layers of tissue in their walls, similar to veins in the cardiovascular system. The inner lining, the **endothelial** layer, covers the valves, which **regulate flow of lymph**. Unlike the cardiovascular system, there is no organ acting as a pump to push lymph through the vessels, but forward pressure is applied to the lymph by various mechanisms, including **squeezing of the vessels by external structures like skeletal**

muscle/intrinsic contractility of the smooth muscle of lymphatic vessel walls. As vessels progressively unite and become wider and wider, eventually they empty into the biggest lymph vessels of all, the **thoracic duct and the right lymphatic duct**. The first one of these drains the **right side of the body above the diaphragm**. The second drains the **lower part of the body and the upper left side above the diaphragm**.

9. and 10.

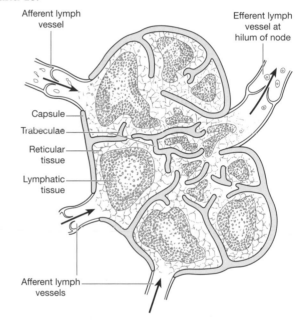

Afferent lymph vessel

Efferent lymph vessel at hilum of node

Capsule
Trabeculae
Reticular tissue
Lymphatic tissue

Afferent lymph vessels

Figure 6.2

11. c.   **12.** a.   **13.** d.   **14.** b.

15. Literally, 'cell eating', the ingestion of unwanted or foreign cells or particles by the body's defence cells, with the intention of destroying or neutralizing them.

16. Malignant cells; infected cells; microbes; inhaled particles; cell debris; worn out cells; damaged cells.

17. They are broken down by enzymes.

18. Sometimes they are broken down chemically but if the cell does not have the enzymes it needs to destroy them, the material may remain indefinitely in the tissues and cause problems, for example inhaled asbestos fibres in the lung.

19. Table 6.1 Characteristics of lymph nodes, spleen and thymus

Spleen	Thymus	Lymph node
Largest lymphatic organ	Maximum weight usually 30–40 g	Size from pin head to almond sized
Lies immediately below the diaphragm	Lies immediately behind the sternum	Distributed throughout lymphatic system
Stores blood	Secretes the hormone thymosin	Phagocytoses cellular debris
Oval in shape	Made up of two narrow lobes	Bean-shaped
Synthesizes red blood cells in the fetus	T-lymphocytes mature here	Site of multiplication of activated lymphocytes
Red blood cells destroyed here	At its maximum size at puberty	Filters lymph

20. c.   **21.** a.   **22.** c.   **23.** b.

7 The nervous system

ANSWERS

1. Brain, spinal cord.

2. and 3. See Figure 7.1.

4. and 5. See Figure 7.2.

6. Myelinated neurones have nodes of Ranvier, non-myelinated neurones do not. One Schwann cell surrounds the axons of many non-myelinated neurones.

7. a. Cell bodies; b. nuclei; c. tracts; d. afferent; e. axons; f. ganglia; g. efferent.

8. Transmission of the **action potential**, or impulse, is due to movement of **ions** across the nerve cell membrane. In the resting state the nerve cell membrane is **polarized** due to differences in the concentrations of ions across the plasma membrane. This means that there is a different electrical charge on each side of the membrane, which is called the resting **membrane potential**. At rest the charge outside the cell is **positive** and inside it is **negative**. The principal ions involved are **sodium** and **potassium**. In the resting state there is a continual tendency for these ions to diffuse down their **concentration gradients**. During the action potential, sodium ions flood **into** the neurone causing **depolarization**. This is followed by **repolarization** when potassium ions move **out of** the neurone. In myelinated neurones the insulating properties of the **myelin sheath** prevent the movement of ions across the membrane where this is present. In these neurones, impulses pass from one **node of Ranvier** to the next and transmission is called **saltatory conduction**. In unmyelinated fibres impulses are conducted by the process called **simple propagation**. Impulse conduction

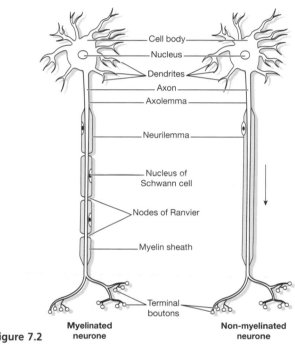

Cell body
Nucleus
Dendrites
Axon
Axolemma
Neurilemma
Nucleus of Schwann cell
Nodes of Ranvier
Myelin sheath
Terminal boutons

Myelinated neurone   **Non-myelinated neurone**

Figure 7.2

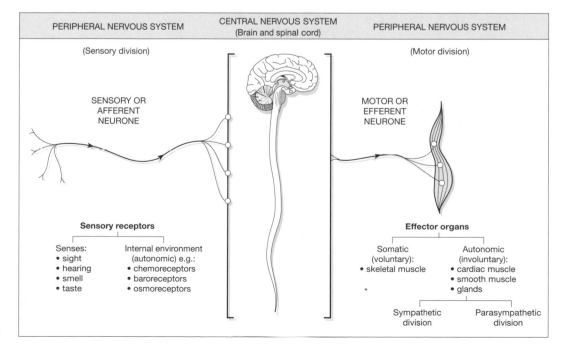

PERIPHERAL NERVOUS SYSTEM   CENTRAL NERVOUS SYSTEM (Brain and spinal cord)   PERIPHERAL NERVOUS SYSTEM

(Sensory division)   (Motor division)

SENSORY OR AFFERENT NEURONE

MOTOR OR EFFERENT NEURONE

Sensory receptors

Senses:
• sight
• hearing
• smell
• taste

Internal environment (autonomic) e.g.:
• chemoreceptors
• baroreceptors
• osmoreceptors

Effector organs

Somatic (voluntary):
• skeletal muscle

Autonomic (involuntary):
• cardiac muscle
• smooth muscle
• glands

Sympathetic division   Parasympathetic division

Figure 7.1

is faster when the mechanism of transmission is **saltatory conduction** than when it is **simple propagation**. The diameter of the neurone also affects the rate of impulse conduction: the **larger** the diameter, the faster the conduction.

9., 10. and 11.

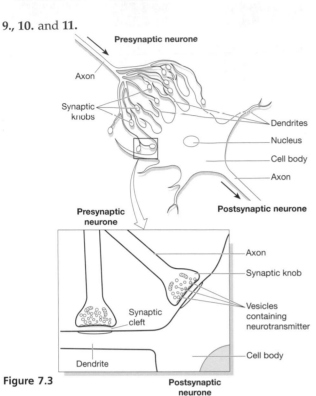

Figure 7.3

12. The region where a nerve impulse passes from one neurone to another is called the **synapse**. The distal end of the presynaptic neurone breaks up into minute branches known as **synaptic knobs/terminal boutons**. These are in close proximity to the dendrites and cell bodies of the **postsynaptic neurone**. The space between them is the **synaptic cleft**. In the ends of the presynaptic neurones are spherical structures called **synaptic vesicles** containing chemicals known as the **neurotransmitter**. When the action potential depolarizes the presynaptic membrane, the chemicals in the membrane-bound packages are released into the synaptic cleft by the process of **exocytosis**. The chemicals released then move across the synaptic cleft by **diffusion**. They act on specific areas of the postsynaptic membrane called **receptors** causing **depolarization**.

13. a. Astrocytes; b. microglia; c. oligodendrocytes; d. astrocytes; e. ependymal cells; f. oligodendrocytes; g. astrocytes.

14. Protects the brain from potentially toxic substances and chemical variations in the blood.

15. Table 7.1 Characteristics of the meninges

	Dura mater	Arachnoid mater	Pia mater
Consists of two layers of fibrous tissue	✓		
Consists of fine connective tissue			✓
A delicate serous membrane		✓	
The subdural space lies between these two layers	✓	✓	
Surrounds the venous sinuses	✓		
The subarachnoid space separates these two layers		✓	✓
Forms the filum terminale			✓
CSF is found in the space between these two layers		✓	✓
Equivalent to the periosteum of other bones	✓		

16.

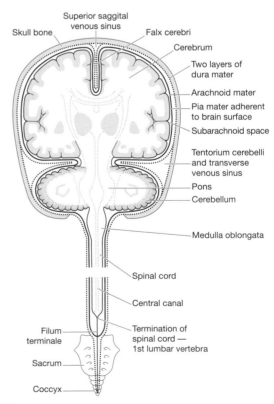

Figure 7.4

17. and 18.

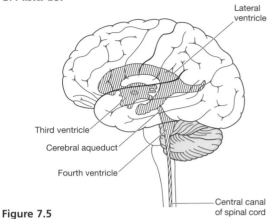

Lateral ventricle

Third ventricle

Cerebral aqueduct

Fourth ventricle

Central canal of spinal cord

Figure 7.5

19. b., c., d.   **20.** a., b., d.   **21.** d.   **22.** b.

23. Supports the brain in the cranial cavity, maintains uniform pressure around the brain and spinal cord, protects the brain and spinal cord by acting as a shock absorber between the brain and cranial bones, keeps the brain and spinal cord moist and may allow exchange of substances between CSF and nerve cells.

24.

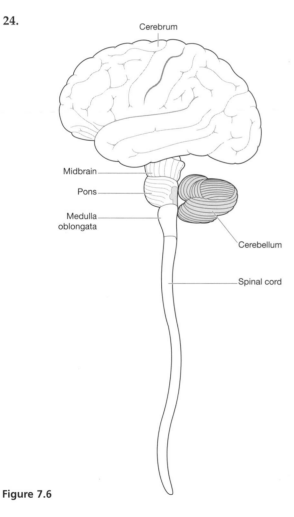

Cerebrum

Midbrain

Pons

Medulla oblongata

Cerebellum

Spinal cord

Figure 7.6

25. This is the largest part of the brain and is divided into left and right **cerebral hemispheres**. Deep inside, the two parts are connected by the **corpus callosum**, which consists of **white** matter. The superficial layer of the cerebrum is known as the **cerebral cortex** and consists of nerve **cell bodies** or grey matter. The deeper layer consists of nerve **fibres** and is **white** in colour. The cerebral cortex has many furrows and folds that vary in depth. The exposed areas are the convolutions or **gyri** and they are separated by **sulci**, also known as **fissures**. These convolutions increase the **surface area** of the cerebrum.

26.

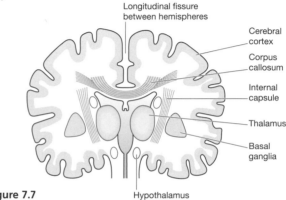

Longitudinal fissure between hemispheres

Cerebral cortex

Corpus callosum

Internal capsule

Thalamus

Basal ganglia

Hypothalamus

Figure 7.7

27. Mental activities, e.g. memory, learning, reasoning; sensory perception; initiation and control of skeletal muscle contraction.

28.

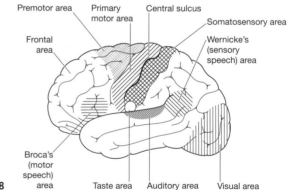

Premotor area

Primary motor area

Central sulcus

Somatosensory area

Frontal area

Wernicke's (sensory speech) area

Broca's (motor speech) area

Taste area

Auditory area

Visual area

Figure 7.8

29. The primary motor area lies in the **frontal** lobe immediately anterior to the **central** sulcus. The cell bodies are **pyramid-shaped** and stimulation leads to contraction of **skeletal** muscle. Their nerve fibres pass downwards through the **internal capsule** to the **medulla** where they cross to the opposite side then descend in the **spinal cord**. These neurones are the upper motor neurones. They synapse with the lower motor neurones in the spinal cord and lower motor neurones terminate at a **neuromuscular junction**. This means that the motor area of the right hemisphere controls skeletal muscle movement on **the left side** of the body.

In the motor area of the cerebrum, body areas are represented **upside down** and the proportion of the cerebral cortex that represents a particular part of the body reflects its **complexity of movement**.

Broca's area lies in the **frontal** lobe and controls the movements needed for **speech**. The right hemisphere is dominant in **left-handed** people.

The frontal area is situated in the **frontal** lobe and is thought to be involved in one's **character**.

30. a. Sensory speech area; b. gustatory area; c. auditory area; d. olfactory area; e. visual area; f. olfactory area; g. auditory area; h. gustatory area and olfactory area; i. visual area; j. auditory area; k. visual area.

31. c.   **32.** a., b., d.   **33.** a., c.   **34.** d.   **35.** a., d.

36. b.   **37.** d.   **38.** c.

39. Insertion of a cannula into the subarachnoid space below the spinal cord (i.e. below the 2nd lumbar vertebra) to measure CSF pressure and/or obtain a sample of CSF.

40. a. Origin – spinal cord, destination – thalamus; b. origin – cerebral cortex, destination – spinal cord.

41. Table 7.2 Characteristics of the motor and sensory pathways of the spinal cord

	Motor pathways	Sensory pathways
Impulses travel towards the brain		✓
The extrapyramidal tracts are an example of these	✓	
Consist of two neurones	✓	
Contain afferent tracts		✓
Their fibres pass through the internal capsule	✓	
Impulses from proprioceptors travel via these pathways		✓
Are involved in fine movements	✓	
Are involved in movement of skeletal muscles	✓	
Impulses follow activation of receptors in the skin		✓
Impulses travel away from the brain	✓	
May consist of either two or three neurones		✓

42., 43. and **44.**

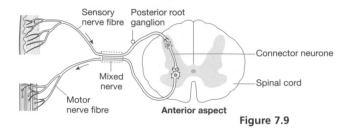

Figure 7.9

45. Within the peripheral nervous system there are **31** pairs of spinal nerves and **12** pairs of cranial nerves. These nerves are composed of either **sensory** nerve fibres conveying afferent impulses to **the brain** from **sensory** organs, or **motor** nerve fibres that transmit efferent impulses from **the brain** to **effector** organs. Some nerves, known as **mixed** nerves contain both types of fibres.

46. It is a site where spinal nerves are regrouped before going on to their destination, meaning that damage to one spinal nerve does not cause loss of function of an area.

47.

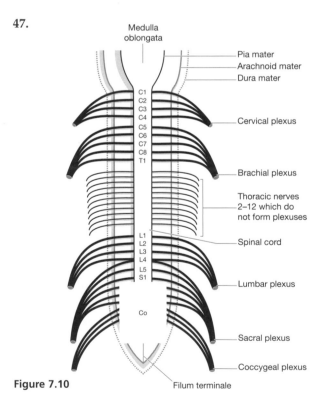

Figure 7.10

48. and 49.

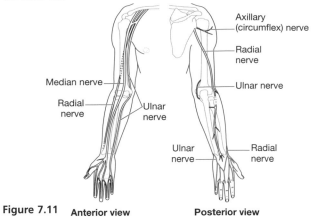

Figure 7.11 **Anterior view**   **Posterior view**

Axillary (circumflex) nerve

Radial nerve

Ulnar nerve

Median nerve

Radial nerve

Ulnar nerve

Ulnar nerve

Radial nerve

50. and 51.

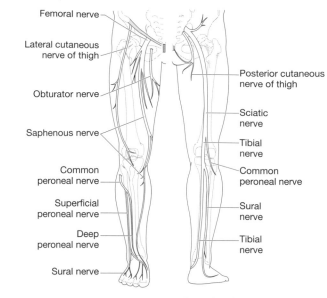

Femoral nerve

Lateral cutaneous nerve of thigh

Obturator nerve

Saphenous nerve

Common peroneal nerve

Superficial peroneal nerve

Deep peroneal nerve

Sural nerve

Posterior cutaneous nerve of thigh

Sciatic nerve

Tibial nerve

Common peroneal nerve

Sural nerve

Tibial nerve

Figure 7.12   **Anterior view**   **Posterior view**

52. a. Intercostal;
   b. phrenic;
   c. sciatic;
   d. pudendal;
   e. pudendal.

53., 54. and 55.

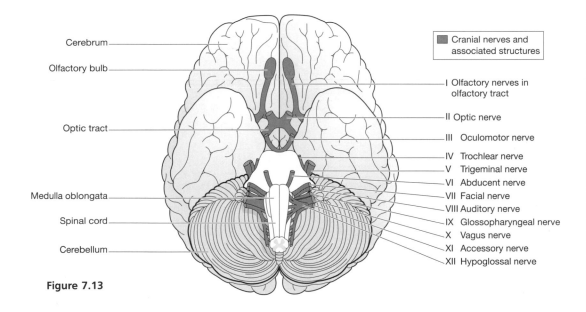

Cerebrum

Olfactory bulb

Optic tract

Medulla oblongata

Spinal cord

Cerebellum

Cranial nerves and associated structures

I Olfactory nerves in olfactory tract
II Optic nerve
III Oculomotor nerve
IV Trochlear nerve
V Trigeminal nerve
VI Abducent nerve
VII Facial nerve
VIII Auditory nerve
IX Glossopharyngeal nerve
X Vagus nerve
XI Accessory nerve
XII Hypoglossal nerve

Figure 7.13

56. and 57. Table 7.3 The cranial nerves and their functions

Number	Name	Function	Type
I	Olfactory	Sense of smell	Sensory
II	Optic	Sense of sight, balance	Sensory
III	Oculomotor	Moving the eyeball, focusing, regulating the size of the pupil	Motor
IV	Trochlear	Movement of the eyeball	Motor
V	Trigeminal	Chewing, sensation from the face	Mixed
VI	Abducent	Movement of the eye	Motor
VII	Facial	Sense of taste, movements of facial expression	Mixed
VIII	Vestibulocochlear	Maintaining balance, sense of hearing	Sensory
IX	Glossopharyngeal	Secretion of saliva, sense of taste, movement of pharynx	Mixed
X	Vagus	Movement and secretion in GI tract, heart rate	Mixed
XI	Accessory	Movement of the head, shoulders and larynx	Motor
XII	Hypoglossal	Movement of the tongue	Motor

58. b., c., d.   **59.** a., d.

60. c.   **61.** b.

62. b.   **63.** a.

64. Smooth muscle, cardiac muscle, glands.

65. Sympathetic, parasympathetic.

66. a. F; b. F; c. T; d. F; e. T; f. F; g. F; h. T.

67. Represented by the dotted lines on Figure 7.14.

68., 69. and **70.** See Figure 7.14

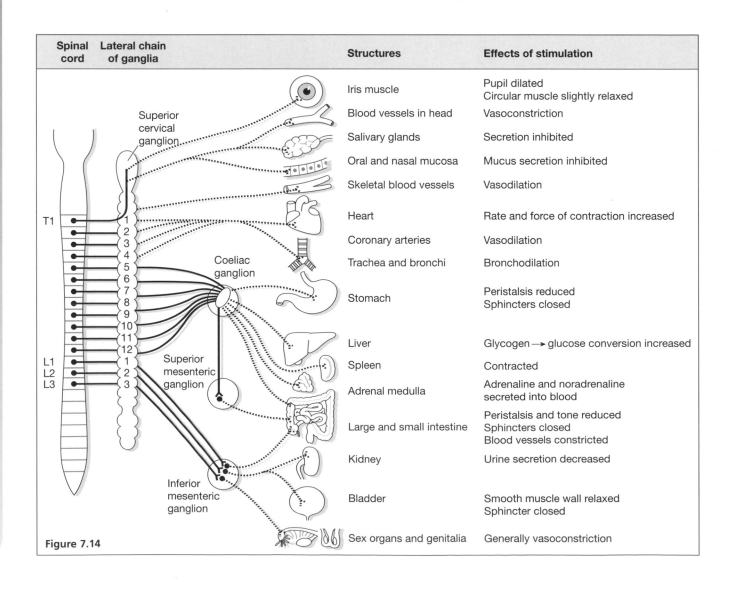

Figure 7.14

71. Represented by the dotted lines on Figure 7.15.

72. In other organs, the cell bodies of parasympathetic postganglionic neurones lie in the wall of the structure supplied and therefore the postganglionic neurone is very small.

73. and **74.**

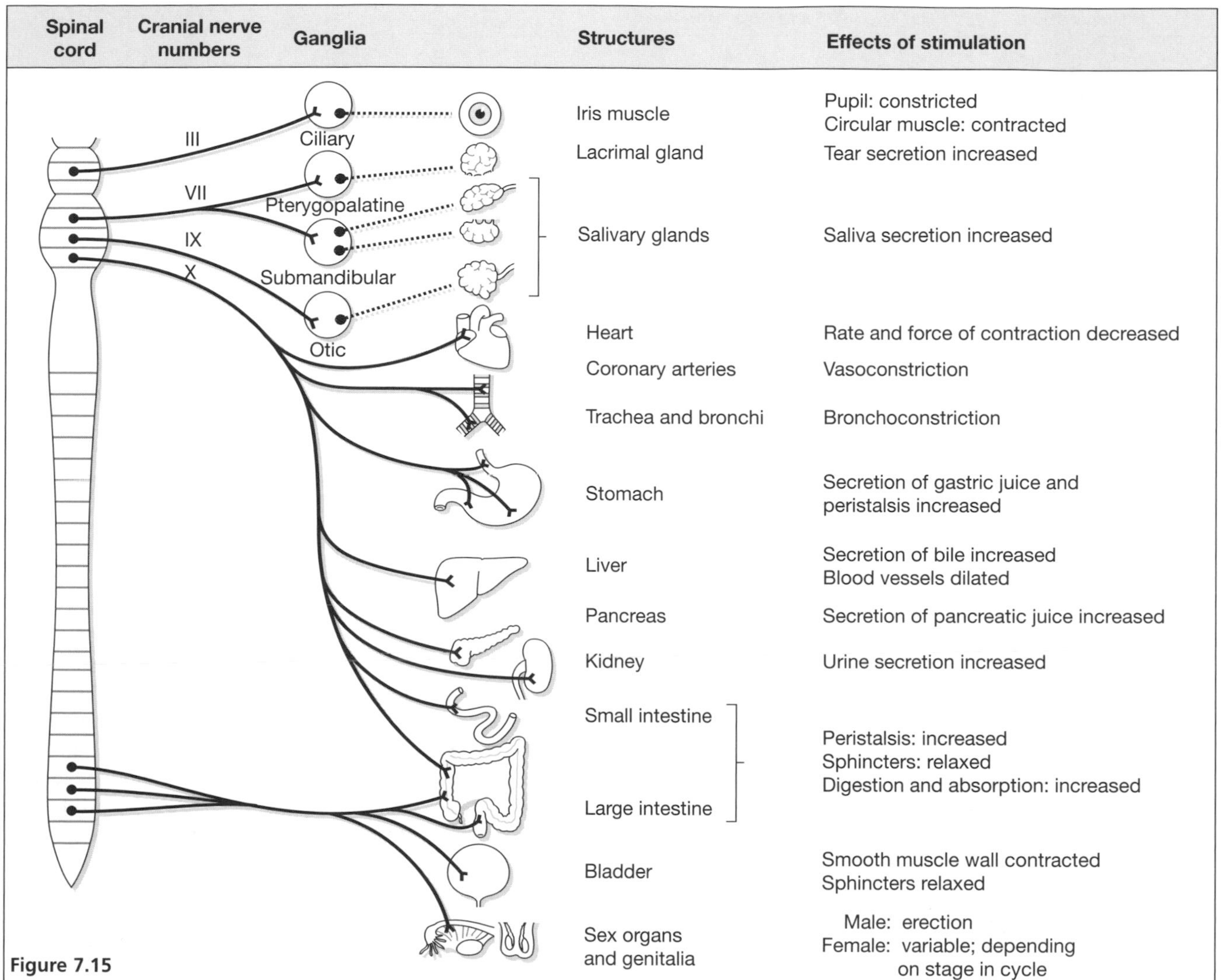

Spinal cord	Cranial nerve numbers	Ganglia	Structures	Effects of stimulation
	III	Ciliary	Iris muscle	Pupil: constricted / Circular muscle: contracted
	VII	Pterygopalatine	Lacrimal gland	Tear secretion increased
	IX	Submandibular	Salivary glands	Saliva secretion increased
	X	Otic		
			Heart	Rate and force of contraction decreased
			Coronary arteries	Vasoconstriction
			Trachea and bronchi	Bronchoconstriction
			Stomach	Secretion of gastric juice and peristalsis increased
			Liver	Secretion of bile increased / Blood vessels dilated
			Pancreas	Secretion of pancreatic juice increased
			Kidney	Urine secretion increased
			Small intestine	Peristalsis: increased / Sphincters: relaxed / Digestion and absorption: increased
			Large intestine	
			Bladder	Smooth muscle wall contracted / Sphincters relaxed
			Sex organs and genitalia	Male: erection / Female: variable; depending on stage in cycle

Figure 7.15

8 The special senses

1. and 2.

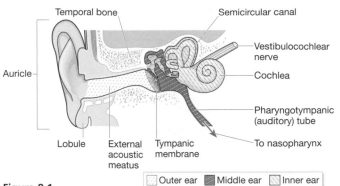

Figure 8.1

3.

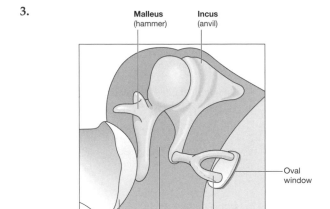

Figure 8.2

6. and 7.

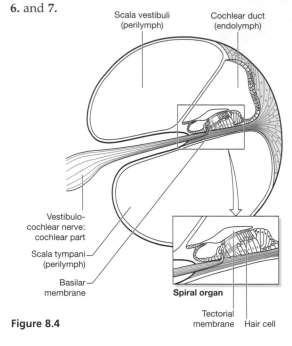

Figure 8.4

8. A sound produces **waves/vibrations** in the air. The auricle **collects** and **directs** them along the **auditory canal** to the **tympanic membrane**. The vibrations are **transmitted** and **amplified** through the middle ear by movement of the **(auditory) ossicles**. At its medial end, movement of the **stapes** in the **oval** window sets up fluid waves in the **perilymph** of the scala vestibuli. Most of this pressure is transmitted into the **cochlear duct** resulting in a corresponding fluid wave in the

4. and 5.

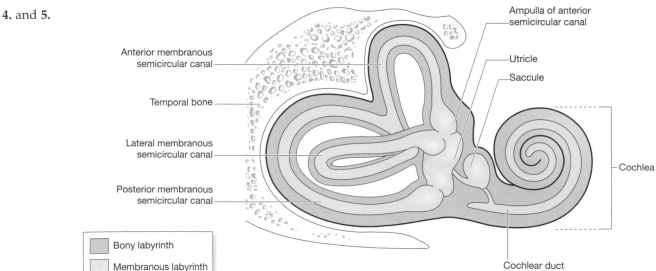

Figure 8.3

endolymph. This stimulates the auditory receptors in the **hair** cells in the organ of hearing, **the spiral organ (of Corti)**. Stimulation of the auditory receptors results in the generation of **nerve impulses** that travel to the brain along the **cochlear/auditory** part of the **vestibulocochlear** nerve. The fluid wave is extinguished by vibration of the membrane of the **round** window.

9., 10. and **11.**

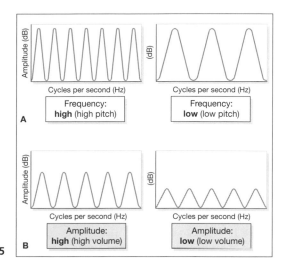

Figure 8.5

12. The organs involved with balance are found in the **inner** ear. They are the three **semicircular** canals, one in each plane of space, and the vestibule, which comprises two parts, the **saccule** and the utricle. The canals, like the cochlea, are composed of an outer bony wall and inner membranous ducts. The membranous ducts contain **endolymph** and are separated from the bony wall by **perilymph**. They have dilated portions near the vestibule called ampullae containing hair cells with sensory nerve endings between them. Any change in the position of the head causes movement in the endolymph and perilymph. This causes stimulation of the hair cells and nerve impulses are generated. These travel in the vestibular part of the vestibulocochlear nerve to the **cerebellum** via the **vestibular** nucleus. Perception of body position occurs because the cerebrum coordinates impulses from the eyes and proprioceptors in addition to those from the cerebellum.

13. and **14.**

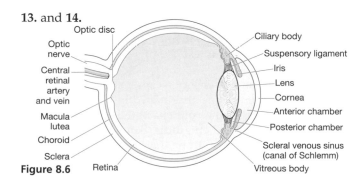

Figure 8.6

15.

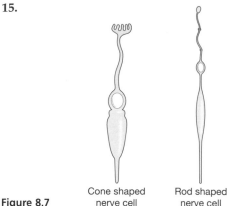

Figure 8.7

16. The anterior segment of the eye is incompletely divided into the **anterior** and **posterior** chambers by the **iris**. Both chambers contain **aqueous fluid** secreted into the **posterior** chamber by the **ciliary glands**. It circulates in front of the **lens** and through the **pupil** into the **anterior** chamber and returns to the circulation through the **scleral venous sinus**. As there is continuous production and drainage, the intraocular pressure remains fairly constant. The structures in the front of the eye including the **cornea** and the **lens** are supplied with nutrients by the **aqueous fluid**. The posterior segment of the eye lies behind the **lens** and contains the **vitreous body**. It has the consistency of **jelly** and provides sufficient intraocular pressure to keep the eyeball from collapsing.

17.

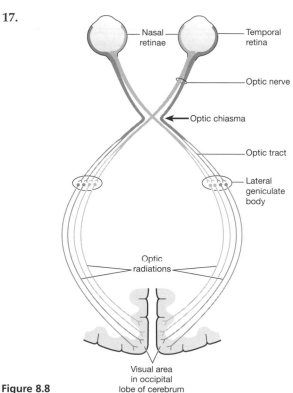

Figure 8.8

18. c.   **19.** c.   **20.** c.   **21.** c.

22.

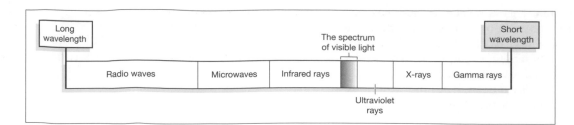

Figure 8.9

23., 24. and 25.

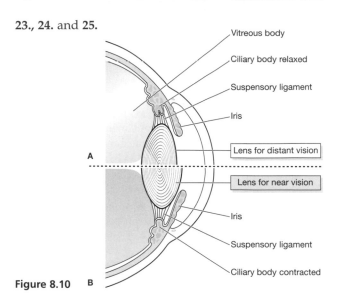

Figure 8.10

29. and 30.

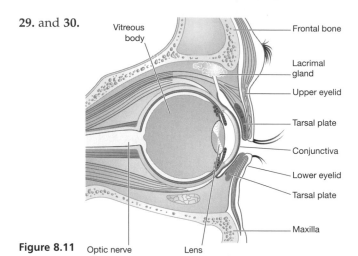

Figure 8.11

26. The amount of light entering the eye is controlled by the **size** of the pupils. In a bright light they are **constricted** and in darkness they are **dilated**. The iris consists of two layers of smooth muscle – contraction of the circular fibres causes **constriction** of the pupil while contraction of the radiating fibres causes **dilation**. The autonomic nervous system controls the size of the pupil – sympathetic stimulation causes **dilation** while parasympathetic stimulation causes **constriction** of the pupil.

27. Constriction of the pupils, convergence of the eyeballs, changing the power of the lens.

28. Table 8.1 Actions of the extrinsic muscles of the eye

Extrinsic muscle	Action
Medial rectus	Rotates the eyeball inwards
Lateral rectus	Rotates the eyeball outwards
Superior rectus	Rotates the eyeball upwards
Inferior rectus	Rotates the eyeball downwards
Superior oblique	Rotates the eyeball downwards and outwards
Inferior oblique	Rotates the eyeball upwards and outwards

31. Water, mineral salts, antibodies, lysozyme.

32. Washing away irritants; the bactericidal enzyme lysozyme prevents infection; the oily secretion from the tarsal glands delays evaporation and prevents drying of the conjunctiva; nourishment of the cornea.

33. All odorous materials give off **volatile** molecules that are carried into the nose in the inhaled air and stimulate the olfactory **chemoreceptors**. When currents of air are carried to the **roof of the nasal cavity** the smell receptors are stimulated setting up impulses in the olfactory nerve endings. These pass through the cribriform plate of the **ethmoid bone** to the olfactory bulb. Nerve fibres that leave the olfactory bulb form the olfactory tract. This passes posteriorly to the olfactory lobe of the **cerebrum or cerebral cortex** where the impulses are interpreted and odour perceived.

34. Absence of the sense of smell.

35. Perception of a particular smell decreases and stops after a few minutes of exposure.

36. Taste buds contain sensory receptors called **chemoreceptors**. They are situated in the papillae of the **tongue** and in the epithelia of the tongue, **soft palate, pharynx** and **epiglottis**. Some of the taste buds have hair-like **microvilli** on their free border projecting towards tiny pores in the epithelium. Sensory receptors are stimulated by chemicals

dissolved in **saliva** and **nerve impulses** are generated when stimulation occurs. These are conducted to the brain where taste is perceived by the **taste/gustatory** area in the **parietal** lobe of the cerebral cortex.

37. and 38.

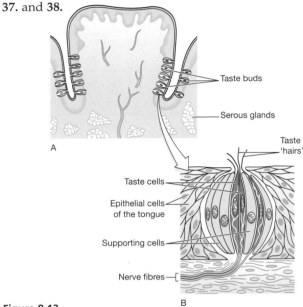

Figure 8.12

39. Sweet, salt, sour, bitter.

40. An abnormal curvature of part of the cornea or lens prevents focusing on the retina, resulting in blurred vision.

41. Nearsightedness – the eyeball is too short resulting in focusing of near images behind the retina.

42. Farsightedness – the eyeball is too long causing a far image to be focused in front of the retina.

43.

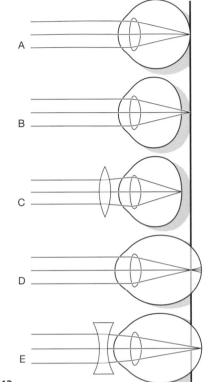

Figure 8.13

9 The endocrine system

ANSWERS

1.

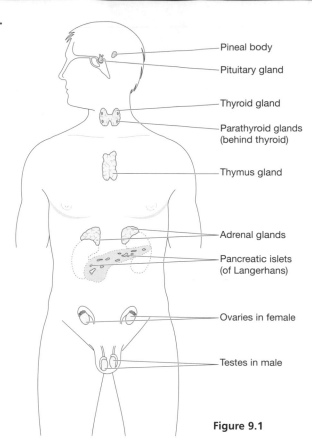

- Pineal body
- Pituitary gland
- Thyroid gland
- Parathyroid glands (behind thyroid)
- Thymus gland
- Adrenal glands
- Pancreatic islets (of Langerhans)
- Ovaries in female
- Testes in male

Figure 9.1

2. Four.

3. There are two embedded in the posterior surface of each lobe of the thyroid gland.

4. A hormone is formed in one organ that **secretes** it into the **bloodstream** which then transports it to its **target organ**. When a hormone arrives at its site of action, it binds to specific molecular groups on the cell membrane called the **receptor**. Homeostasis of the **internal** environment is maintained partly by the **autonomic** nervous system and partly by the endocrine system. The former is concerned with **fast** changes while those that involve the endocrine system are **slow** and more precise adjustments. Chemically, hormones fall into two groups: **protein based** and **lipid based**. Hormones in the first group are **water** soluble and include **insulin, glucagon** and **adrenaline** (epinephrine). The latter group includes **steroids** and **thyroid hormones**.

5. Table 9.1 Anatomy of the pituitary gland

Posterior lobe of the pituitary gland	Neurohypophysis
Anterior lobe of the pituitary gland	Adenohypophysis
Connects the pituitary gland to the hypothalamus	Pituitary stalk
Composed of glandular tissue	Anterior lobe of the pituitary
Composed of nervous tissue	Posterior lobe of the pituitary
Part of the pituitary whose function is unknown in humans	Intermediate lobe of the pituitary
Transports blood from the hypothalamus to the anterior pituitary	Pituitary portal system
Situated superiorly to the pituitary gland	Hypothalamus
A hollow in the sphenoid bone	Hypophyseal fossa
A supporting cell of the posterior pituitary	Pituicyte

6. Table 9.2 Summary of the hormones secreted by the anterior pituitary gland

Hormone	Abbreviation	Function
Growth hormone	GH	Regulates metabolism, promotes tissue growth – especially bone
Thyroid stimulating hormone	TSH	Stimulates growth and activity of the thyroid gland
Adrenocorticotrophic hormone	ACTH	Stimulates the adrenal glands to secrete glucocorticoids
Prolactin	PRL	Stimulates milk production in the mammary glands
Follicle stimulating hormone	FSH	Males: stimulates production of sperm in the testes
		Females: stimulates secretion of oestrogen in the ovaries, maturation of ovarian follicles, ovulation
Luteinizing hormone	LH	Males: stimulates secretion of testosterone in the testes
		Females: stimulates secretion of progesterone by the corpus luteum

7. and 8.

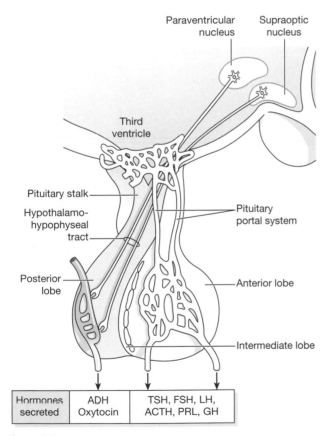

Figure 9.2

9. and 10.

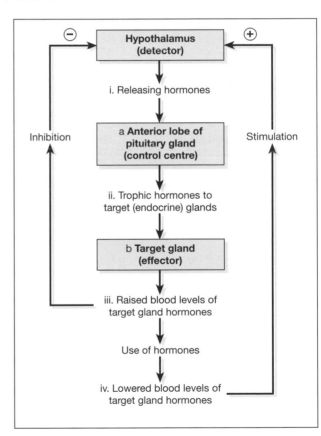

Figure 9.3

11. a., b., c.   **12.** a., b., c.   **13.** d.   **14.** a.

15. a.   **16.** b.   **17.** c., d.   **18.** c.

19. Oxytocin stimulates two target tissues before and after childbirth. These are uterine **smooth muscle** and **myoepithelial cells** of the lactating breast. During childbirth, also known as **parturition**, increasing amounts of oxytocin are released in response to increasing **stimulation** of sensory **stretch receptors** in the **(uterine) cervix** by the baby's head. Sensory impulses are generated and travel to the **hypothalamus** stimulating the **posterior pituitary** to secrete more oxytocin. This **stimulates** the uterus to contract more forcefully moving the baby's head further downwards through the uterine cervix and vagina. The mechanism stops shortly after the baby has been born. This is an example of a **positive** feedback mechanism. After birth oxytocin stimulates **lactation**.

20. Table 9.3 Features of the thyroid gland

The thyroid gland is surrounded by this structure	Capsule
Joins the two thyroid lobes together	Isthmus
Lie against the posterior surface of the thyroid gland	Parathyroid glands
Secrete the hormone calcitonin	Parafollicular cells
Constituent of T_3 and T_4	Iodine
Secreted by the hypothalamus	TRH
Thyroxine	T_4
Precursor of T_3 and T_4	Thyroglobulin
Secreted by the anterior pituitary	TSH
The nerves close to the thyroid gland	Recurrent laryngeal

21.

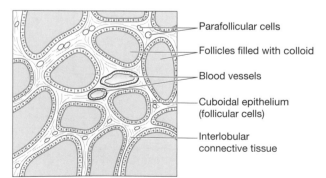

Figure 9.4

22. Table 9.4 Effects of abnormal secretion of thyroid hormones

Body function affected	Hypersecretion of T_3 and T_4	Hyposecretion of T_3 and T_4
Metabolic rate	Increased	Decreased
Weight	Loss	Gain
Appetite	Good	Poor, anorexia
Mental state	Anxious, excitable, restless	Depressed, lethargic, mentally slow
Scalp	Hair loss	Brittle hair
Heart	Tachycardia, palpitations, atrial fibrillation	Bradycardia
Skin	Warm and sweaty	Dry and cold
Faeces	Loose – diarrhoea	Dry – constipation
Eyes	Exophthalmos	None

23.

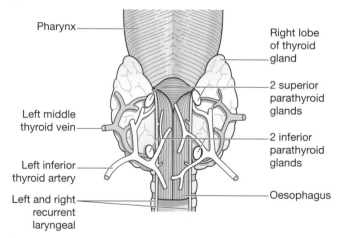

Figure 9.5

24. The parathyroid glands secrete parathyroid hormone (PTH, **parathormone**). Blood calcium levels regulate its secretion. When they **fall**, secretion of PTH is increased and vice versa. The main function of PTH is to **increase** the blood calcium level. This is achieved by **increasing** the amount of calcium absorbed from the small intestine and reabsorbed from the renal tubules. Normal blood calcium levels are needed for muscle **contraction**, blood clotting and nerve impulse transmission.

25. Table 9.5 Features of the adrenal glands

Is essential for life	Cortex
Inner part of the adrenal gland	Medulla
Veins that drain the adrenal glands	Suprarenal
The organs immediately inferior to the adrenal glands	Kidneys
Male sex hormones	Androgens
The lipid that forms the basic structure of adrenocorticoids	Cholesterol
A mineralocorticoid hormone	Aldosterone
A glucocorticoid hormone	Hydrocortisone

26. and **27.** See Figure 9.6.

28. a. alpha (α); b. beta (β); c. delta (δ).

29. a. T; b. F; c. T; d. F; e. F; f. T; g. F; h. T.

30. and **31.** Table 9.6 The effect of insulin and glucagon on metabolic processes

Metabolic pathway	Effect of pathway on metabolism	Stimulated by insulin or glucagon?
Gluconeogenesis	Formation of new sugar from e.g. protein	Glucagon
Lipogenesis	Promoting synthesis of fatty acids and storage of fat	Insulin
Glycogenesis	Increasing conversion of glucose to glycogen	Insulin
Glycogenolysis	Conversion of glycogen to glucose	Glucagon
Lipolysis	Breakdown of triglycerides to fatty acids	Insulin

32. a., b.　　**33.** b., c.　　**34.** d.　　**35.** a., c.

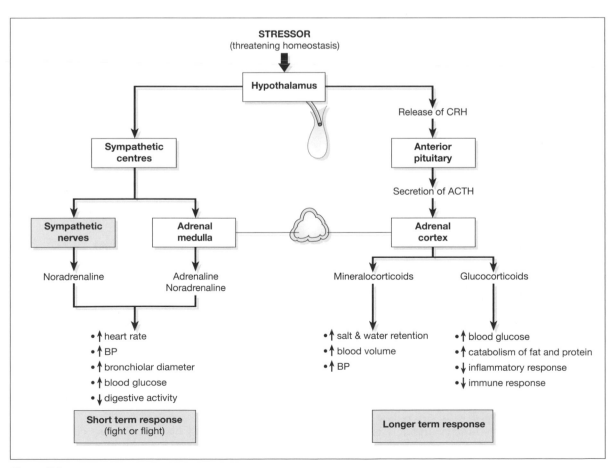

Figure 9.6

10 The respiratory system

ANSWERS

1. and 2.

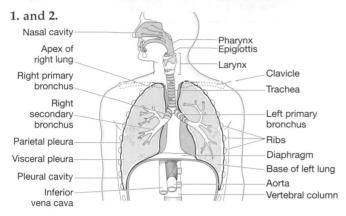

Nasal cavity

Apex of right lung

Right primary bronchus

Right secondary bronchus

Parietal pleura

Visceral pleura

Pleural cavity

Inferior vena cava

Pharynx
Epiglottis

Larynx

Clavicle

Trachea

Left primary bronchus

Ribs

Diaphragm

Base of left lung

Aorta

Vertebral column

Figure 10.1

3. a. Nasal conchae, b. larynx, c. thyroid cartilage, d. epiglottis, e. soft palate, f. tonsils, g. auditory tube.

4.

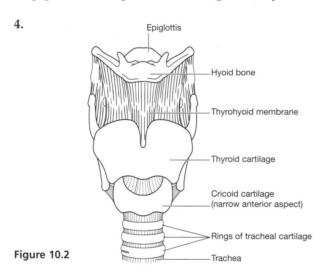

Epiglottis

Hyoid bone

Thyrohyoid membrane

Thyroid cartilage

Cricoid cartilage (narrow anterior aspect)

Rings of tracheal cartilage

Trachea

Figure 10.2

5. The upper respiratory passages carry air in and out of the respiratory system, but they have other functions too. The cells of their mucous membrane have **cilia**, tiny hair-like structures that **beat** in a wave-like motion towards the **mouth**. They carry **mucus**, which has been made by the **goblet** cells in the epithelial layer, and which traps **dirt** and **dust** on its sticky surface. The air is therefore **cleaned** by these mechanisms before it gets into the lungs. As the air passes through the nasal cavity, it is also **warmed** and **moistened** as it passes over the nasal **conchae**, bony projections covered in mucous membrane. The nasal cavity also contains **hair**, which is covered in **mucus**, and acts as a coarse filter for the air passing through. Immune tissue is present in patches called **tonsils**, which make **antibodies** and therefore protect against inhaled antigens. Not only air

passes through the pharynx, but also **food** and **drink**, and the tracheal opening is barricaded against these by the **epiglottis**.

6.

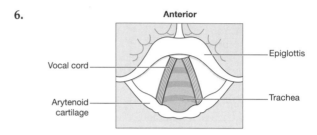

Anterior

Vocal cord

Arytenoid cartilage

Epiglottis

Trachea

Figure 10.3

7. d.   **8.** a.   **9.** a.   **10.** c.   **11.** d.

12.

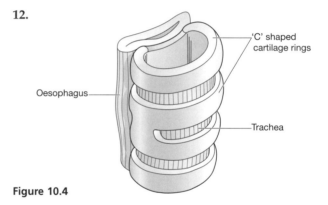

'C' shaped cartilage rings

Oesophagus

Trachea

Figure 10.4

13. C-shaped, with the opening at the back (i.e. lying against the oesophagus).

14. To permit expansion of the oesophagus when swallowing, without obstructing the trachea.

15.

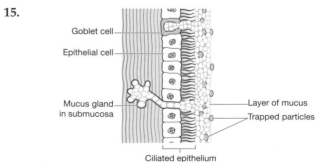

Goblet cell

Epithelial cell

Mucus gland in submucosa

Layer of mucus

Trapped particles

Ciliated epithelium

Figure 10.5

16. Cell A: Ciliated epithelial cell; protects and lines; cilia clear mucus and inhaled particles from the airways. Cell B: Goblet cell; produces sticky mucus that traps inhaled particles.

17. a. Mucus is produced in the upper respiratory tract because this an efficient way of removing dust and dirt from inhaled air. b. Cilia are present in the upper respiratory tract because mucus needs to be swept away from the lungs. c. Cartilage is present in the upper respiratory tract because the airways have to be kept open at all times. d. Elastic tissue is present in the upper respiratory tract because the passageway has to be flexible to allow head and neck movement.

18. Ciliated respiratory epithelium lines the **upper respiratory tract and wider airways only**, and its job is to keep the lungs clean. Cartilage rings support the airway walls; as the airways progressively divide and their diameter decreases, the amount of cartilage present **also decreases**. The smallest airways are called respiratory bronchioles, **and some** gas exchange takes place across their walls. The airways terminate in clusters of microscopic pouches called alveoli; it is here that most gas exchange takes place. The alveolar walls are necessarily very thin: only one cell thick. This layer contains **alveolar cells**, which make surfactant to keep the alveoli from collapsing. Gas exchange occurring across the alveolar walls is called **external** respiration.

19. and **20.**

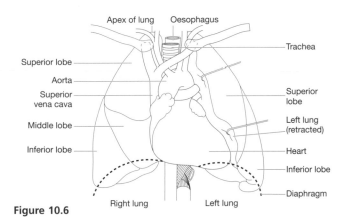

Figure 10.6

21. Mediastinum.

22.

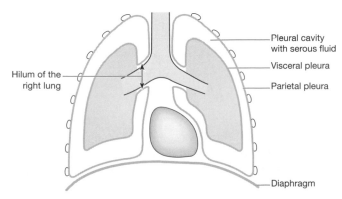

Figure 10.7

23. In the pleural cavity, in between the two layers of the pleural membrane and its function is to allow the lungs to inflate and deflate without friction.

24. a.   **25.** b.   **26.** b.   **27.** a.

28.

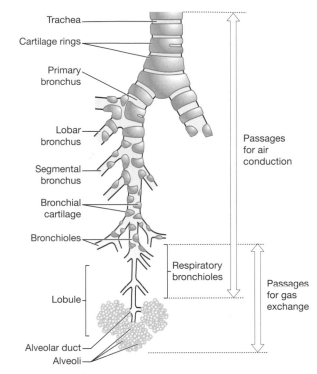

Figure 10.8

29.

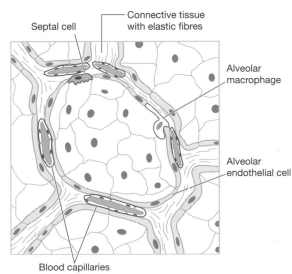

Figure 10.9

30. Cell A: surfactant, septal cell
Cell B: phagocytosis; macrophage

31. Left atrium, left ventricle, aorta, body tissues, right atrium, right ventricle, pulmonary artery, lungs, pulmonary vein.

32. Just before inspiration commences, the diaphragm is **relaxed**; this occurs in the pause between breaths in normal quiet breathing. Inspiration commences. The ribcage moves **upwards** and **outwards** owing to contraction of the **intercostal muscles**. The diaphragm **contracts** and moves **downwards**. This **increases** the volume of the thoracic cavity, and **decreases** the pressure. Because of these changes, air moves **into** the lungs, and the lungs **inflate**. Inspiration has taken place.

Unlike inspiration, expiration is usually a **passive** process because it requires no **muscular effort**. So, following the end of inspiration, the diaphragm **relaxes** and moves back into its resting position. The ribcage moves **downwards** and **inwards**, because the **intercostal muscles** have relaxed. This **decreases** the volume of the thoracic cavity, and so **increases** the pressure within it. Air therefore now moves **out of** the lungs and they **deflate**. There is now a rest period before the next cycle begins.

33. c.   **34.** a.   **35.** b., c.   **36.** d.

37.

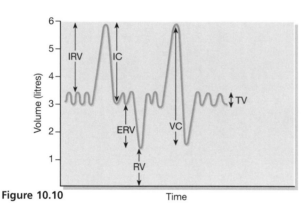

Figure 10.10

a. Tidal volume; b. vital capacity; c. inspiratory capacity; d. residual volume; e. inspiratory reserve volume; f. expiratory reserve volume.

38. IC is 3000 ml; IRV is 2500 ml.

39. 4800 ml.

40. 3770 ml.

41. Both residual volume and vital capacity are fixed measures, determined by individual anatomical and physiological constraints, and are unaffected by exercise.

42. Exchange of gases in the lung; oxygen leaves the alveoli and enters the blood, and carbon dioxide leaves the blood and enters the lung, both gases moving down their pressure gradients.

43. Exchange of gases in the tissues; oxygen leaves the blood and enters the tissues, and carbon dioxide leaves the tissues and enters the blood, both gases moving down their pressure gradients.

44. It is very thin, and has a large surface area.

45. There are very many capillaries, and the blood cells move through them in single file.

46. External respiration.

47, 48, 49

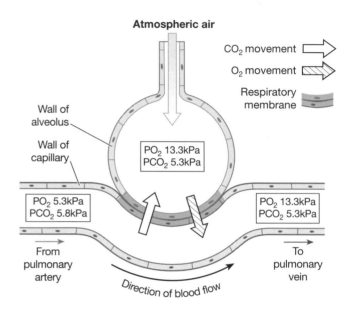

Figure 10.11

50. Internal respiration.

51, 52

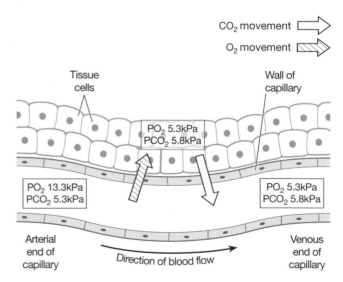

Figure 10.12

53. b.

54. d.

55. a. Carbon dioxide diffuses from the body cells into the bloodstream because PCO_2 is lower in the capillary than the tissues. b. Tissue levels of oxygen are lower than blood levels because body cells are continuously using oxygen. c. Oxygen diffuses out of the capillary because PO_2 is lower in the tissues than in the bloodstream. d. The arterial end of the capillary is higher in oxygen than the venous end because as the blood flows through the tissues it releases oxygen into the cells.

56. a. CO_2, b. CO_2, c. O_2, d. CO_2, e. O_2, f. both, g. O_2, h. O_2, i. CO_2.

57.

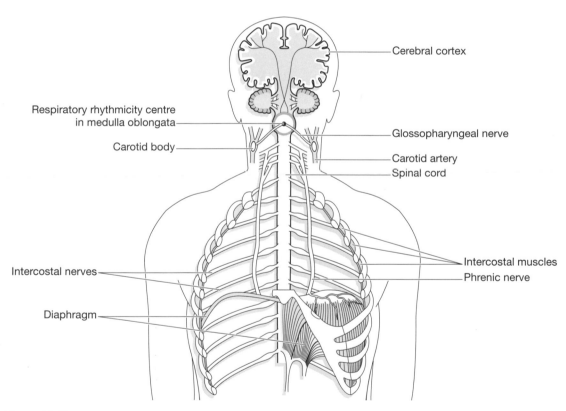

Cerebral cortex

Respiratory rhythmicity centre in medulla oblongata

Glossopharyngeal nerve

Carotid body

Carotid artery

Spinal cord

Intercostal nerves

Intercostal muscles

Phrenic nerve

Diaphragm

Figure 10.13

58. Table 10.1 Causes of increased/decreased respiratory effort

Stimulus	Increases respiratory effort	Decreases respiratory effort
Fever	✓	
Pain	✓	
Sedative drugs		✓
Acidification of the CSF	✓	
Sleep		✓
Exercise	✓	
High blood [H^+]	✓	
Increased alkalinity of the blood		✓
Increased pH of the CSF		✓
Hypoxaemia	✓	
Hypercapnia	✓	
Stimulation of the respiratory centre	✓	
Decreased CO_2 excretion	✓	

59. d.

60. a., c.

61. d.

62. a.

11 Nutrition

ANSWERS

1. Carbohydrates, proteins, fats, vitamins, minerals, water.

2. and 3.

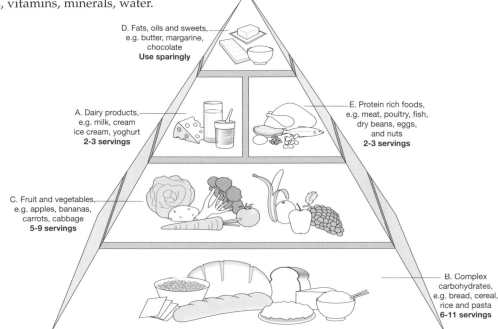

Figure 11.1

D. Fats, oils and sweets,
e.g. butter, margarine,
chocolate
Use sparingly

A. Dairy products,
e.g. milk, cream
ice cream, yoghurt
2-3 servings

E. Protein rich foods,
e.g. meat, poultry, fish,
dry beans, eggs,
and nuts
2-3 servings

C. Fruit and vegetables,
e.g. apples, bananas,
carrots, cabbage
5-9 servings

B. Complex
carbohydrates,
e.g. bread, cereal,
rice and pasta
6-11 servings

4. a., c., d.   **5.** a., b.   **6.** c., d.   **7.** a., d.

8. Those that must be eaten in the diet because the body cannot sythesize them.

9. Those that the body can synthesize for itself.

10. A protein source containing all essential amino acids in correct proportions.

11. Growth and repair of body tissues; an alternative energy source when carbohydrates and fats are not available; building blocks for synthesis of enzymes, plasma proteins, antibodies, enzymes.

12. The three elements that make up fat are **carbon, hydrogen** and **oxygen**. Fats are usually divided into two groups: **saturated** fats are found in foods from animal sources, such as **meat**, **fish** and **eggs**. The second group, the **unsaturated** fats, are found in vegetable oils. Fat (adipose) tissue is laid down under the skin, where it acts as an **insulator**. It is also found around the kidneys, where its function is to **support** these organs. Fat depots in the body are important as **energy** sources. Certain hormones, such as **steroids** e.g. **cortisone**, are synthesized from the fatty precursor **cholesterol**, also found in the cell membrane. In addition, certain substances are absorbed with fat in the intestine, a significant example being the **fat soluble vitamins**, which are essential for health despite being required only in tiny amounts. Fats in a meal have the direct effect of **slowing** gastric emptying and **delaying** the return of a feeling of hunger.

13. Table 11.1 Vitamin sources

Vitamin	Main sources
A	Cream, egg yolk, liver, fish oil, milk, cheese, butter
B_1 (thiamine)	Nuts, egg yolk, yeast, liver, legumes, meat, cereal germ
B_2 (riboflavine)	Yeast, green vegetables, milk, liver, egg yolk, cheese
Folate (folic acid)	Liver, kidney, leafy green vegetables, yeast
Niacin	Liver, cheese, yeast, eggs, fish, nuts, whole cereal
B_6 (pyridoxine)	Egg yolk, peas, beans, yeast, meat, liver
B_{12} (cyanocobalamin)	Liver, meat, eggs, milk, fermented products
Pantothenic acid	Many foods
Biotin	Yeast, egg yolk, liver, kidney, tomatoes
C	Fresh citrus fruit
D	Animal fats, e.g. eggs, butter, cheese, fish oils
E	Nuts, egg yolk, wheat germ, whole cereal, milk, butter
K	Fish, liver, leafy green vegetables and fruit

14. a. Vitamins C and E; b. vitamin C; c. vitamin A; d. vitamin B_6; e. vitamin A; f. vitamins B_1, B_2 and biotin; g. vitamin K; h. vitamins B_6, B_{12}, folate (folic acid); i. pantothenic acid, vitamin B_6; j. vitamin D; k. niacin; l. vitamin B_{12}.

15. Because vitamin A is a fat soluble vitamin, its absorption can be reduced if **bile** secretion into the gastrointestinal tract is lower than normal. The first sign of deficiency is **night blindness**, and this may be followed by **conjunctival ulceration**. On the other hand, the B complex vitamins are water soluble. Most of them are involved in **biochemical release of energy**. Thiamine deficiency is associated with **beriberi**, and niacin inadequacy leads to **pellagra**. Folic acid is required for **DNA** synthesis, and is therefore often prescribed as a supplement in pregnancy. Deficiency of vitamin B_{12} typically leads to **megaloblastic** anaemia, because it is needed for DNA synthesis, and is usually associated with lack of **intrinsic factor** in the gastrointestinal tract.

    Vitamin C is needed for **connective tissue synthesis**. One of the first signs of deficiency of this vitamin is therefore loosening of the teeth, due to **defective gum tissue**. Vitamin C is destroyed by **heat**.

    Lack of vitamin D causes **osteomalacia** in adults, and **rickets** in children. Vitamin E deficiency results in **haemolytic** anaemia, because the **cell membrane** of red blood cells is damaged.

    Vitamin K deficiency leads to problems with **blood coagulation**.

16. Table 11.2 Functions of minerals

17. a., b.   18. a., b.   19. a., c., d.

20. a.   21. a., b., c., d.   22. a, d.

23. Non-starch polysaccharide

24. Bulking diet and satisfying appetite; stimulating peristalsis of the intestines; attracting water that softens faeces; increases frequency of defaecation and prevents constipation; reduces incidence of certain gastrointestinal disorders.

25. Fruit, vegetables, whole cereals.

26. Men – 70%; women – 60%.

	Calcium	Phosphate	Sodium	Potassium	Iron	Iodine
Needed for haemoglobin synthesis					✓	
Used in thyroxine manufacture						✓
Most abundant cation outside cells			✓			
99% of body stock is found in bones	✓					
Most abundant cation inside cells				✓		
May be added to table salt						✓
Vitamin D is needed for use	✓	✓				
Involved in muscle contraction	✓		✓	✓		
Used to make high-energy ATP		✓				
Needed for normal blood clotting	✓					
Required for hardening of teeth	✓	✓				
Needed for normal nerve transmission			✓	✓		

12 | The digestive system

ANSWERS

1. and **2.** The large intestine includes all regions of the colon and the rectum (see Fig. 12.1)

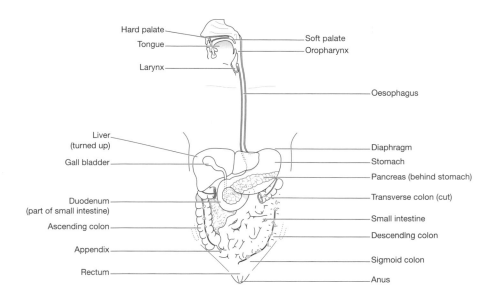

Hard palate
Tongue
Larynx
Liver (turned up)
Gall bladder
Duodenum (part of small intestine)
Ascending colon
Appendix
Rectum
Soft palate
Oropharynx
Oesophagus
Diaphragm
Stomach
Pancreas (behind stomach)
Transverse colon (cut)
Small intestine
Descending colon
Sigmoid colon
Anus

Figure 12.1

3. An enzyme is a chemical catalyst, usually a protein, which speeds up a chemical reaction without itself being changed or used up; one enzyme molecule can therefore catalyse large numbers of reactions.

4. Ingestion, propulsion, digestion, absorption and elimination.

5. Mechanical digestion is the physical squeezing, chopping or cutting of food in the gastrointestinal system, e.g. chewing by the teeth and churning in the stomach. Chemical digestion involves the breaking down of the molecules that make up the food into smaller ones that can be absorbed; this is accomplished by the gastrointestinal enzymes.

6. Table 12.1 Organs of the alimentary tract and accessory organs

Organs of alimentary tract	Accessory organs
Mouth	Liver
Oesophagus	Gall bladder
Stomach	Pancreas
Small intestine	Sublingual glands
Large intestine	Submandibular glands
Rectum and anus	Parotid glands

7. and 8.

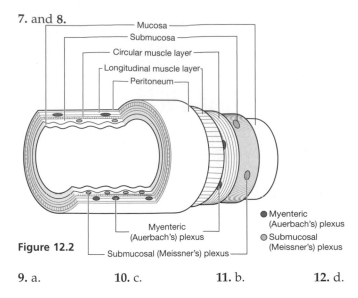

Figure 12.2

9. a.   **10.** c.   **11.** b.   **12.** d.

13., 14. and **15.** This is columnar epithelium with goblet cells. Mucus lubricates the foodstuffs and protects the lining of the gastrointestinal tract.

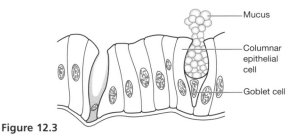

Figure 12.3

16. In areas where secretion and absorption occur, e.g. stomach and small/large intestine.

17. d.   **18.** b.   **19.** d.   **20.** b.

21. and **22.** A = incisors, B = canines, C = premolars, D = molars; A and B: cutting and biting, C and D: grinding and chewing.

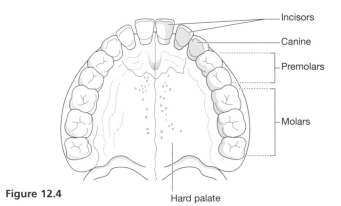

Figure 12.4

23. and 24.

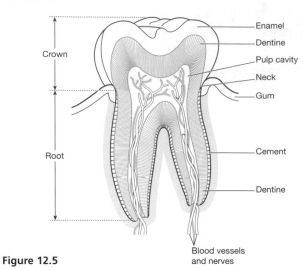

Figure 12.5

Cement – a bone-like substance that fixes the tooth in its socket.
Dentine – layer of the tooth lying below the enamel and surrounding the pulp cavity.
Enamel – very hard outer layer of the tooth that forms the crown.

25. Nerves, blood and lymph vessels.

26. Eight premolars (four at the bottom and four at the top), and four molars.

27.

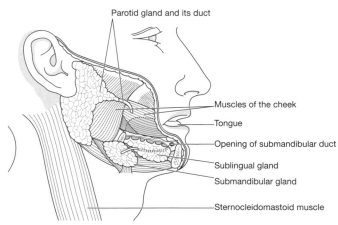

Figure 12.6

28. Parotid gland – duct opens into the mouth next to the second upper molar.
Submandibular gland – duct opens onto the floor of the mouth on each side of the frenulum.
Sublingual gland – numerous small ducts open into the floor of the mouth.

29.

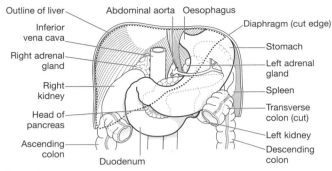

Figure 12.7

30.

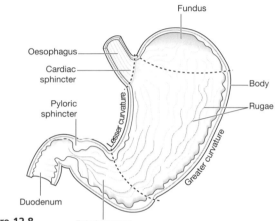

Figure 12.8

31. There are three layers of muscle in the stomach, oblique, circular and longitudinal fibres, not two as found elsewhere.

32. This contributes to the efficient churning action of the stomach.

33. a. Hydrochloric acid, intrinsic factor; b. hydrochloric acid; c. mucus; d. hydrochloric acid; e. pepsinogens; f. pepsinogens; g. pepsinogens; h. intrinsic factor; i. hydrochloric acid; j. mucus; k. pepsinogens; l. hydrochloric acid.

34. b.   **35.** b.   **36.** d.   **37.** c.

38. a. True; b. Chemical digestion in the stomach includes the action of **pepsin**, an enzyme that acts on proteins and breaks them down to smaller polypeptides. c. True; d. The stomach has **little** absorptive function; its environment is too acidic, and absorption cannot occur until the food has been neutralized in the intestines. e. True; f. Absorption of iron takes place **in the small intestine**; the acid environment of the stomach solubilizes iron salts, an essential step in iron absorption. g. True; h. The stomach regulates flow of liquidized food into the next part of the digestive tract, the duodenum, through the **pyloric** sphincter.

39. Table 12.2 Characteristics of the duodenum, jejunum and ileum

	Duodenum	Jejunum	Ileum
Longest portion of the small intestine			✓
Curves around the head of the pancreas	✓		
Vitamin B$_{12}$ is absorbed here			✓
About 25 cm long	✓		
Middle section		✓	
Ends at the ileocaecal valve			✓
Flow in is regulated by the pyloric sphincter	✓		
Most digestion takes place here	✓		
About 2 m long		✓	
Flow from here enters the large intestine			✓
Bile passes into this section	✓		
The pancreas passes its secretions into this section	✓		
Villi present here	✓	✓	✓
Most absorption takes place here		✓	

40. and **41.** (See Figure 12.9.) Mucosa forms the villi.

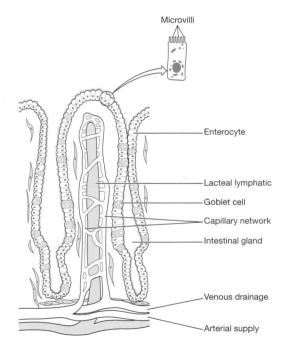

Figure 12.9

42. Digested fats.

43. Aggregated lymphatic follicles (Peyer's patches).

44. On a daily basis, the intestine secretes about **1500 ml** of intestinal juices, and its contents are **between 7.8 and 8.0**. In the small intestine, chemical digestion is completed and the end products are absorbed. The main enzyme secreted by the enterocytes is enterokinase, which **activates enzymes from the pancreas**. However, other enzymes from accessory structures are passed into the **duodenum** as well.

The pancreas secretes **amylase**, which is important in reducing large sugar molecules to **disaccharides**. In addition, pancreatic lipase breaks down fats into **fatty acids and glycerol**, which can be absorbed in the intestine. The third major nutrient group, the proteins, are broken down to **dipeptides** by pancreatic **trypsin and chymotrypsin**. Pancreatic juice is also rich in **bicarbonate** ions, important in neutralizing the acid chyme from the stomach.

Bile is made in the **liver**, stored in the **gall bladder**, and enters the intestine via the **hepatopancreatic sphincter**. It has a role to play in fat digestion by breaking fats into **tiny droplets**. This increases the action of lipases on the fat.

Even after the multiple digestive actions of these enzymes, the digested proteins and carbohydrates are still not in a readily absorbable form, and digestion is completed by enzymes made by the **enterocytes**. Thus, the final stage of protein digestion produces **amino acids** and the final stage of carbohydrate digestion produces **monosaccharides**.

45. d.   **46.** b.   **47.** a., d.   **48.** b.

49.

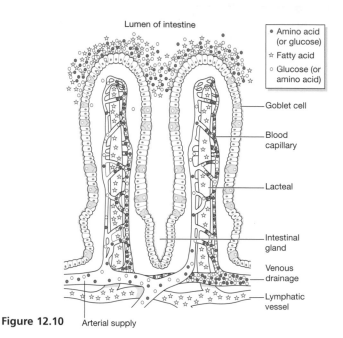

Figure 12.10

50. A, D, E and K in the lacteal (fat soluble); B and C in the blood.

51. Active transport.

52. Glucose, amino acids, fatty acids, glycerol, disaccharides, dipeptides, tripeptides.

53. See Figure 12.11.

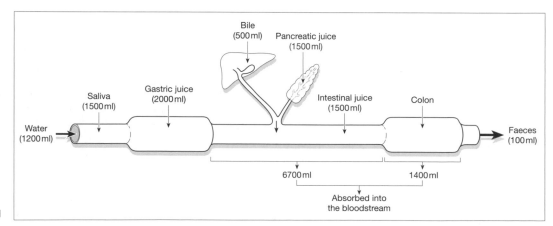

Figure 12.11

54. b.   **55.** a.   **56.** d.   **57.** c.   **61.** Diaphragm.

58.

62.

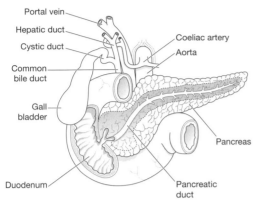

Figure 12.12

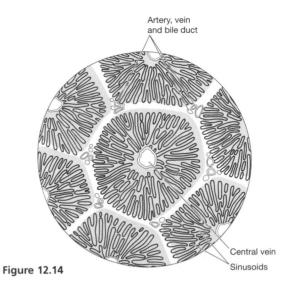

Figure 12.14

59. Table 12.3 Functions of the pancreas

Exocrine functions	Endocrine functions
Secretion of enzymes	Secretion of insulin
Passes secretions into duodenum	Control of blood sugar levels
Secretions leave via the pancreatic duct	Secretion of hormones
Role is in digestion	Substances are passed directly into blood
Synthesis takes place in pancreatic alveoli	Secretion of glucagon
Secretions include amylase, lipase and proteases	Synthesis takes place in the pancreatic islets

60.

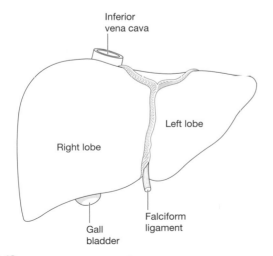

Figure 12.13

63. The arterial supply is from the hepatic artery and nourishes the liver tissues; the venous supply is the hepatic portal vein which is bringing blood from the intestines, to be purified before being returned to the venous circulation.

64. The liver is involved in the metabolism of carbohydrates; it converts glucose to **glycogen** for storage; the hormone that is important for this is **insulin**. In the opposite reaction, glucose is released to meet the body's energy needs and the important hormone for this is **glucagon**. This action of the liver maintains the blood sugar levels within close limits. Other metabolic processes include the formation of waste, including **urea** from the breakdown of protein, and **uric acid** from the breakdown of nucleic acids. Transamination is the process by which **new amino acids** are made from **carbohydrates**. Proteins are also made here; two important groups of proteins, found in the blood, are the **clotting proteins** and the **plasma proteins**.

    The liver detoxifies many ingested chemicals, including **alcohol** and **drugs**. It also breaks down some of the body's own products, such as **hormones**. Red blood cells and other cellular material such as microbes are broken down in the **Kupffer** cells. It synthesizes vitamin **A** from **carotene**, a provitamin found in plants such as carrots, and stores it, along with other vitamins. The liver is also the main storage site of **iron** (essential for haemoglobin synthesis).

    The liver makes **bile**, which is stored in the gall bladder and important in digestion of **fats**. Bile salts are important for **emulsifying fats** in the small intestine, and are themselves reabsorbed from the gut and returned to the liver in the **blood**. This is called the **enterohepatic** circulation, and helps to conserve the body's store of bile salts. Bilirubin is released when **red blood cells** are broken down (this occurs mainly in the **spleen** and the **liver**). Bilirubin is not very soluble, so to increase its water solubility so that it can be excreted in the bile, it is conjugated with **glucuronic acid**. On its passage through the intestine, it is converted by bacteria to **stercobilin**, which is excreted in the faeces; some is, however, reabsorbed and excreted in the urine as **urobilinogen**. If levels of bilirubin in the blood are high, its yellow colour is seen in the tissues as **jaundice**.

65., 66. and **67.**

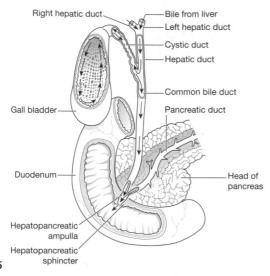

Figure 12.15

68. c.   **69.** a.   **70.** c.   **71.** c.

72. Catabolism is the breaking down of large molecules into smaller ones, often to release stored energy.

73. Anabolism is the synthesis of large molecules from smaller ones, usually requiring energy.

74. A kilocalorie is the amount of heat (energy) needed to raise the temperature of 1 litre of water by 1 degree Celsius. It is equivalent to 4.184 kilojoules.

75. c.   **76.** d.   **77.** a.   **78.** b.   **79.** b., c., d.   **80.** c.

81. and **82.**

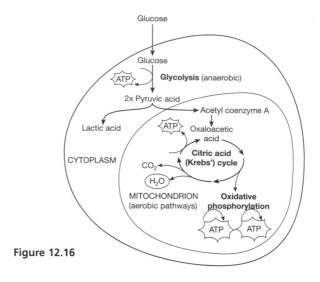

Figure 12.16

83. and **84.**

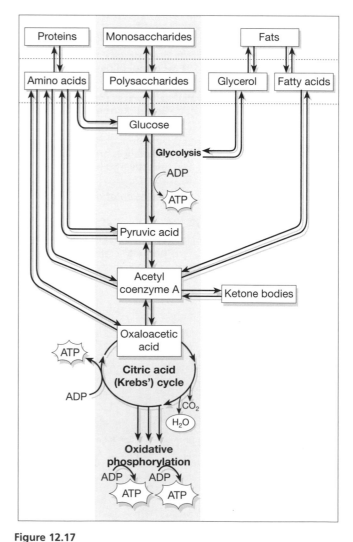

Figure 12.17

85. Oxygen.

13 The urinary system

ANSWERS

1. and 2.

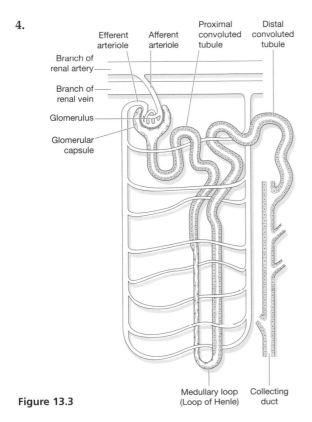

Figure 13.1

Inferior vena cava
Right adrenal gland
Right kidney
Duodenum
Right ureter
Left adrenal gland
Left kidney
Pancreas
Aorta
Left ureter
Bladder

3.

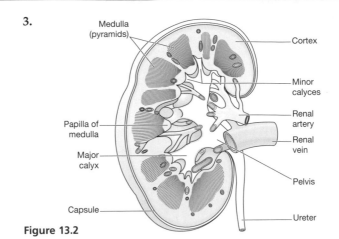

Figure 13.2

Medulla (pyramids)
Papilla of medulla
Major calyx
Capsule
Cortex
Minor calyces
Renal artery
Renal vein
Pelvis
Ureter

5.

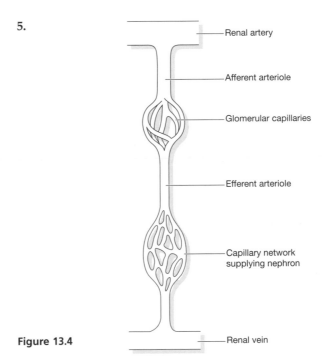

Figure 13.4

Renal artery
Afferent arteriole
Glomerular capillaries
Efferent arteriole
Capillary network supplying nephron
Renal vein

4.

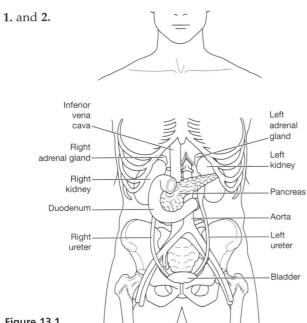

Figure 13.3

Efferent arteriole
Afferent arteriole
Proximal convoluted tubule
Distal convoluted tubule
Branch of renal artery
Branch of renal vein
Glomerulus
Glomerular capsule
Medullary loop (Loop of Henle)
Collecting duct

6. b , c.   **7.** a., b., c., d.   **8.** d.   **9.** b., c., d.

10. d.   **11.** c.

12. Filtration, reabsorption, secretion.

13. and **14.**

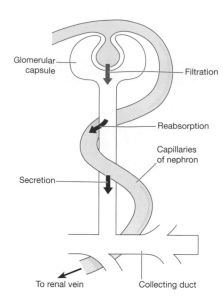

Figure 13.5

15. Table 13.1 Characteristics of normal urine

Colour	Amber
Specific gravity	1020–1030
pH	6 (normal range = 4.5–8)
Average daily volume	1000–1500 ml

16. Table 13.2 Normal constituents of glomerular filtrate and urine

Constituent of blood	Presence in glomerular filtrate	Presence in urine
Water	Normal	Normal
Sodium	Normal	Normal
Potassium	Normal	Normal
Glucose	Normal	Abnormal
Urea	Normal	Normal
Creatinine	Normal	Normal
Proteins	Abnormal	Abnormal
Uric acid	Normal	Normal
Red blood cells	Abnormal	Abnormal
White blood cells	Abnormal	Abnormal
Platelets	Abnormal	Abnormal

17. Water is excreted through the lungs in **saturated expired air**, through the skin as **sweat** and via the kidneys as the main constituent of **urine**. Of these three, the most important in controlling fluid balance are the **kidneys**. The minimum urinary output required to excrete the body's waste products is about **500 ml** per day. The volume in excess of this is controlled mainly by the hormone **ADH (antidiuretic hormone)**. Sensory nerve cells, called **osmoreceptors**, detect changes in the osmotic pressure of the blood. They are situated in the **hypothalamus**. When the osmotic pressure increases, secretion of ADH is **increased** and water is **reabsorbed** by the distal collecting tubules and collecting ducts. These actions result in the osmotic pressure of the blood being **decreased**. This control system maintains osmotic pressure of the blood within a narrow range and is known as a **negative feedback** system.

18. Sodium (g)
Potassium (e)
Water (h)
Increased (d)
Volume (i)
Vasoconstriction (c)
Renin (a)
ACE (angiotensin converting enzyme) (b)
Aldosterone (f)

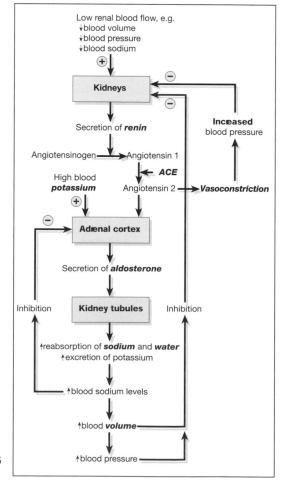

Figure 13.6

19. (j) Stimulates; (k) inhibits; (l) inhibits; (m) inhibits.

20. Table 13.3 The sites of production of substances that influence the composition of urine

Substance	Site of production
Antidiuretic hormone	Posterior lobe of the pituitary gland
Aldosterone	Adrenal cortex
Angiotensin converting enzyme	Lungs and proximal convoluted tubules
Renin	Afferent arteriole of the nephron
Angiotensinogen	Liver
Atrial natriuretic peptide	Atrial walls in the heart

21. The ureters propel urine from the **kidneys** to the bladder by the process of **peristalsis**. Each ureter is about **25–30 cm** long and **3 mm** in diameter. They enter the bladder at an **oblique** angle that prevents **reflux/backflow** of urine into the ureter as the bladder fills and during **micturition**.

22. a.   23. b.   24. b., c.   25. d.

26.

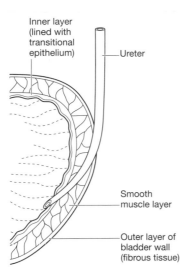

Figure 13.7

27. and 28.

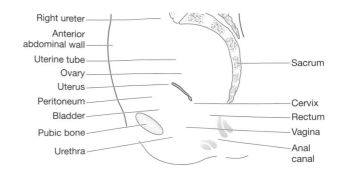

A

B

Figure 13.8

29. The bladder acts as a **reservoir** for urine. When empty, its shape resembles a **pear** and it becomes more **oval** as it fills. The posterior surface is the **base** and the bladder opens into the urethra at its lowest point, the **neck**. The bladder wall is composed of three layers. The outer layer is composed of **connective tissue** and contains **blood** and **lymphatic** vessels. The muscular layer is formed by **smooth** muscle arranged in **three** layers. Collectively this is called the **detrusor** and when it contracts the bladder **empties**. The inner layer is the **mucosa** and it is lined with **transitional epithelium**. Three orifices on the posterior bladder wall form the **trigone**. The two upper openings are formed when each **ureter** enters the bladder and the lower one is the opening of the **urethra**.

30. d.   31. c.   32. b.   33. c.   34. a., b., c.

35. As the bladder fills and becomes distended, receptors in the wall are stimulated by **stretching**. In infants this initiates a **spinal reflex** and micturition occurs as nerve impulses to the bladder cause **contraction** of the **detrusor** muscle and **relaxation** of the **internal** urethral sphincter. When the nervous system is fully developed the micturition reflex is stimulated but sensory impulses pass upwards to the **brain**. By conscious effort, the reflex can be **over-ridden**. In addition to the processes involved in infants, there is **voluntary** relaxation of the **external** urethral sphincter.

36. Secretion of excessive volumes of urine.

37. Presence of sugar in urine.

38. Excessive thirst.

39. Presence of ketones in urine.

40. Plasma proteins; erythrocytes; leukocytes.

41. When glucose levels in the filtrate exceed the transport maximum of the kidneys no more glucose can be reabsorbed. It is therefore excreted in the urine together with large volumes of water. This leads to polyuria, polydipsia and dehydration.

42. It becomes excessive due to the absence of ADH.

43. They reduce blood pressure (antihypertensive agents).

14 The skin

ANSWERS

1., 2. and **3.**

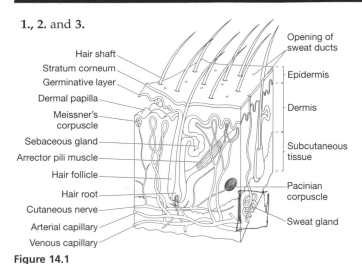

Hair shaft
Stratum corneum
Germinative layer
Dermal papilla
Meissner's corpuscle
Sebaceous gland
Arrector pili muscle
Hair follicle
Hair root
Cutaneous nerve
Arterial capillary
Venous capillary

Opening of sweat ducts
Epidermis
Dermis
Subcutaneous tissue
Pacinian corpuscle
Sweat gland

Figure 14.1

4. c.   **5.** c.   **6.** a., b., d.   **7.** b., d.

8. Table 14.1 Sensory receptors and their stimuli

Sensory receptor	Stimulus
Meissner's corpuscle	Light pressure
Pacinian corpuscle	Deep pressure
Free nerve ending	Pain

9. a. Sensory nerve endings; b. conduction; c. vasodilation; d. vitamin D; e. Langerhans cells; f. evaporation; g. absorption; h. convection; i. non-specific defence mechanism.

10. a. Gain; b. Loss; c. Loss; d. Loss; e. Loss; f. Gain; g. Loss; h. Loss.

11. The temperature regulating centre is situated in the **hypothalamus** and is responsive to the temperature of circulating **blood**. When body temperature rises, sweat glands are stimulated by the **autonomic nervous system**. The **vasomotor** centre in the medulla oblongata controls the diameter of small arteries and **arterioles** and therefore the amount of **blood** circulating in the dermis. When body temperature rises the skin capillaries **dilate** and extra blood near the surface increases heat loss by **radiation, convection** and **conduction**. The skin is warm and **pink** in colour. When body temperature falls, arteriolar vasoconstriction conserves heat and the skin is **whiter/paler** and feels cool.

Fever is often the result of **infection**. During this process there is release of chemicals, also called **pyrogens**, from damaged tissue. These chemicals act on the **hypothalamus/temperature regulating centre** which releases prostaglandins that reset the temperature thermostat to a **higher** temperature. The body responds by activating heat promoting mechanisms, e.g. **shivering** and **vasoconstriction**, until the new temperature is reached. When the thermostat is reset to the normal level, heat loss mechanisms are activated. There is vasodilatation and profuse **sweating** until body temperature returns to the normal range again.

12. Table 14.2 Factors affecting the rate of wound healing

	Promote wound healing	Impair wound healing
Systemic factors	Good nutritional status Good health	Infection Impaired immunity or illness
Local factors	Good blood supply	Contaminants

13. Healing that occurs when there is minimal loss of tissue and damaged skin edges are in close proximity.

14. Healing that occurs when there is destruction or loss of large amounts of tissue or when the edges of the wound cannot be brought together.

15. and **16.**

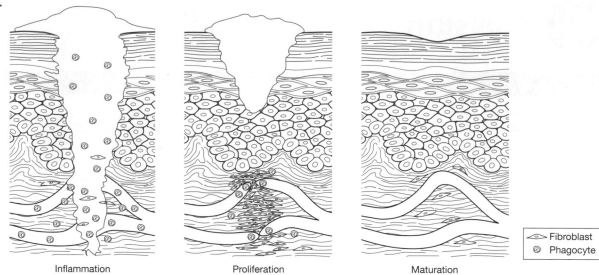

Figure 14.2   Inflammation   Proliferation   Maturation

Fibroblast
Phagocyte

17. b., c.   **18.** a., c.   **19.** a., b., d.   **20.** b.   **21.** a., d.

22. Core body temperature less than 35°C.

23. Vasconstriction occurs to conserve heat and blood supply to the skin is reduced and therefore there is less blood (containing the red pigment haemoglobin) there.

24. As body temperature drops, shivering occurs in an attempt to reverse heat loss. As body temperature decreases further heat loss continues and when heat conserving mechanisms fail, shivering stops.

Resistance and immunity

ANSWERS

1. Defence mechanisms that protect against a wide range of invaders, such as the barrier action of intact skin and the non-selective phagocytic activity of macrophages.

2. Defence mechanisms that operate against one antigen only, such as antibodies to the measles virus.

3. a., b., c.　　　**4.** c.　　　**5.** a.　　　**6.** d.

7. Phagocytosis.

8.

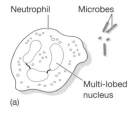
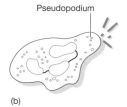
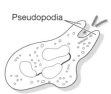
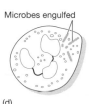

Figure 15.1 (c)　　　(d)

9. a. Neutrophil has been attracted towards invading bacteria; b. neutrophil is extending pseudopodium towards bacteria; c. the pseudopodia begin to encircle bacteria; d. bacteria are engulfed and will be destroyed.

10. and **11.** (See Figure 15.2.)
A. Monocyte, a type of white blood cell, which migrates into the tissues in inflammation and differentiates into macrophages; B. macrophage, derived from a monocyte, a large efficient phagocyte that clears up tissue debris and microbes; C. mast cell, which makes and stores histamine in its cytoplasmic granules; D. neutrophil, a small phagocyte from the blood which is first on the scene in an acute inflammatory reaction.

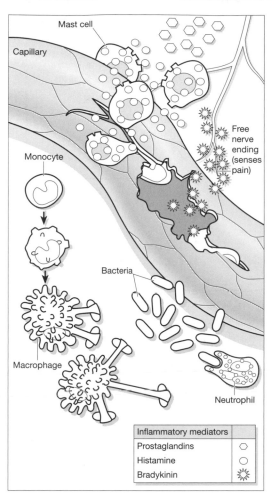

Figure 15.2

12. Redness, swelling, pain, heat, loss of function.

13. c.　　　**14.** d.　　　**15.** b., c.　　　**16.** a., b., c., d.

17. Table 15.1 Summary of some important inflammatory mediators

Substance	Made by	Trigger for release	Main actions
Histamine	Mast cells in tissues and basophils in blood	Binding of antibody to mast cell or basophil plasma membrane	Vasodilation, itch, ↑ vascular permeability, degranulation, smooth muscle contraction (e.g. bronchoconstriction)
Serotonin	Platelets, mast cells and basophils; neurotransmitter in central nervous system	When platelets are activated and when mast cells/basophils degranulate	Vasoconstriction, ↑ vascular permeability
Prostaglandins	Synthesized as required from cell membranes	Many triggers, e.g. drugs, toxins, other mediators, trauma, hormones	Diverse, sometimes opposing, e.g. fever, pain, vasodilation or vasoconstriction, ↑ vascular permeability
Heparin	Liver, mast cells, basophils	When cells degranulate	Anticoagulant, maintaining blood supply to an inflamed area
Bradykinin	Tissues and blood	Blood clotting, trauma, inflammation	Pain, vasodilation

18. a., c.   **19.** b.   **20.** d.   **21.** a.   **22.** d.

23. Table 15.2 Lymphocyte characteristics

Characteristic	T-lymphocyte	B-lymphocyte
Shape of nucleus	Large, single	Large, single
Site of manufacture	Bone marrow	Bone marrow
Site of post-manufacture processing	Thymus gland	Bone marrow
Nature of immunity involved	Cell-mediated	Antibody-mediated
Specific or non-specific defence	Specific	Specific
Production of antibodies	No	Yes (as plasma cells)
Processing regulated by thymosin	Yes	No

24., 25.

Macrophage is a non-specific phagocyte but in the immune response it presents antigenic fraction of antigen to unstimulated T-lymphocytes. Unspecialized T-lymphocytes have been processed to recognize only one antigen but have not yet encountered it; it will be activated by the macrophage showing it the antigen it is educated to look for.

Cytotoxic T-lymphocyte is one type of differentiated T-lymphocyte active in direct cell–cell killing, i.e. any cell that shows the target antigen will be destroyed.

Helper T-lymphocyte synthesizes chemicals to support other cells, and is also needed to interact with B-lymphocytes before B-lymphocytes can be activated to make antibody. Memory T-lymphocyte is long-lived and survives after infection is resolved; it will stimulate a faster and stronger response next time; this is the basis of immunity. Suppressor T-lymphocytes turn off the immune response once the threat has been dealt with.

26. They are all the same, i.e. clonal expansion gives rise to different populations of T-cells that are all specific to the original antigen.

27. Clonal expansion.

28. and 29.

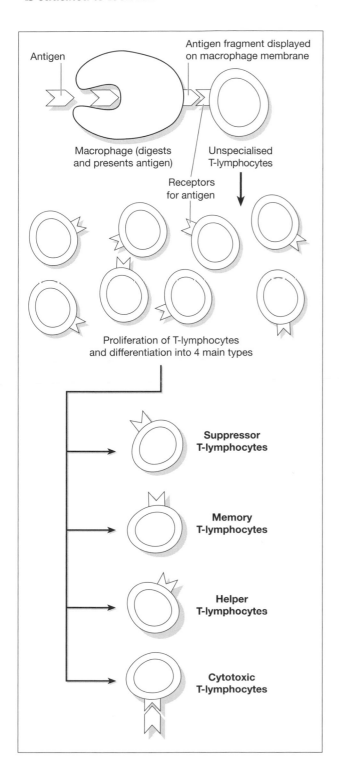

Figure 15.3

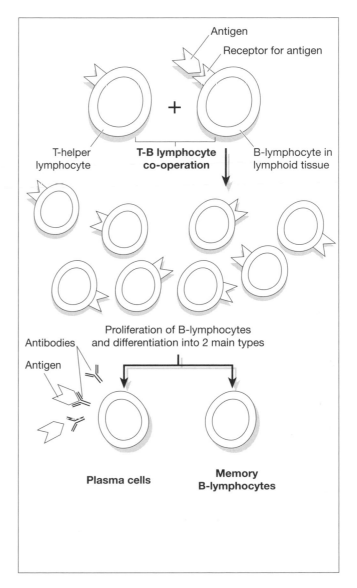

Figure 15.4

28. and 29. *(Cont'd)*

Helper T-lymphocyte is presenting antigen to the B-lymphocyte (i.e. is showing it the antigen it is looking for), and this stimulates the B-lymphocyte to divide and differentiate.

B-lymphocyte has been processed to recognize only one antigen, but has not yet encountered it; it will be activated by the helper T-cell showing it the antigen it is educated to look for.

Memory B-lymphocyte is long-lived and survives after infection is resolved; it will stimulate a faster and stronger response next time; this is the basis of immunity.

Plasma cell is derived from activated B-lymphocytes and makes antibody to the original antigen.

30. T–B lymphocyte co-operation, essential for B-cell activation.

31. They are all the same; activated T lymphocytes only activate the B-cells carrying the same surface receptor as themselves, and so the B-cells make antibody only to the original antigen.

32. a **33.** d **34.** a **35.** d

36. When the body is exposed to an antigen for the first time, the immune response can be measured as antibody levels in the blood after about **2 weeks**; this is the **primary** response. Antibody levels fall thereafter, and do not rise again unless there is a second exposure to the same antigen, which stimulates a **secondary** response, which is different from the first in that it is much **faster** and antibody levels become much **higher**. After having been exposed to an antigen, an individual may develop immunity to it, provided he has produced a population of **memory** cells.

37. Table 15.3 The four types of acquired immunity

Characteristic	Active natural	Active artificial	Passive natural	Passive artificial
An example is a baby's consumption of antibodies in its mother's milk			✓	
Long-lived protection	✓	✓		
Involves production of memory cells	✓	✓		
An example is vaccination		✓		
Short-lived protection			✓	✓
An example is infusion of antibodies				✓
Involves production of antibodies by the individual	✓	✓		
An example is a child catching chickenpox at school	✓			
Specific	✓	✓	✓	✓

16 The musculoskeletal system

ANSWERS

1.

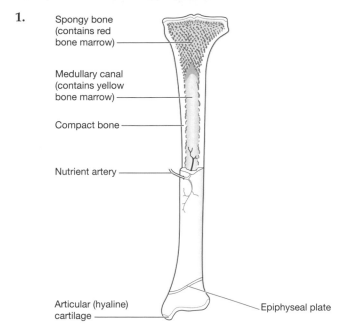

Spongy bone (contains red bone marrow)

Medullary canal (contains yellow bone marrow)

Compact bone

Nutrient artery

Articular (hyaline) cartilage

Epiphyseal plate

Figure 16.1

2. Periosteum.

3. a. Femur, tibia, fibula; b. carpals (wrist); c. vertebrae; d. sternum, ribs; e. patella (knee cap).

4.

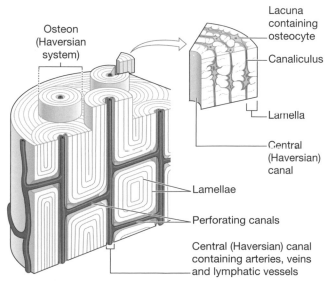

Osteon (Haversian system)

Lacuna containing osteocyte

Canaliculus

Lamella

Central (Haversian) canal

Lamellae

Perforating canals

Central (Haversian) canal containing arteries, veins and lymphatic vessels

Figure 16.2

5. Table 16.1 Characteristics of bone

Spongy bone	Looks like a honeycomb to the naked eye
Osteoblasts	Cells that lay down bone
Osteoclasts	Cells that break down bone
Osteon	Haversian system
Spongy bone	Cancellous bone
Cortical bone	Compact bone
Trabeculae	Form the framework of spongy bone
Chrondroblasts	Cells that lay down cartilage
Osteocytes	Mature osteoblasts
Interstitial lamellae	Remains of old osteons
Lacunae	Spaces between lamellae that contain osteocytes
Red bone marrow	Found mainly in spaces within spongy bone
Flat bones	Develop from membrane models
Sesamoid bones	Develop from tendon models
Long bones	Develop from cartilage models

6. Bone tissue develops in the foetus from **connective tissue** models. This process is called **osteogenesis/ ossification** and is **incomplete** at birth. The main constituent of bone is **calcium salts**, and the organic component is primarily **collagen**. During life, bone growth is stimulated by **thyroxine/oestrogen**, but its density is decreased by **lack of exercise**.

7. and **8.** a. Fossa b. border c. trochanter d. foramen
e. condyle f. meatus g. suture h. fissure i. crest/spine
j. facet k. sinus

S	C					T		T
I	O		C	R	E	S	T	R
N	N		C					O
U	D		A					C
S	Y	F	O	S	S	A		H
	L							A
B	M	E	A	T	U	S		E	N
O				R			S		T
R	F	I	S	S	U	R	E	P	E
D			T				I	R
E		U					N
R		S	F	O	R	A	M	E	N

9. Table 16.2 Types of fractures

Type of fracture	Characteristics
Simple	Bone ends do not protrude through the skin
Compound	Bone ends protrude through the skin
Pathological	Fracture of a bone weakened by disease

10. a.   **11.** b.   **12.** d.   **13.** a.

14. Presence of tissue fragments between the bone ends; poor blood supply; poor alignment of bone ends; mobility of the bone ends.

15. and **16.** (See Figure 16.3.)

17. and **18.** (See Figure 16.4.)

19. a. Palatine; b. maxilla; c. vomer;
d. occipital; e. temporal;
f. sphenoid; g. ethmoid;
h. temporal;
i. occipital; j. lacrimal.

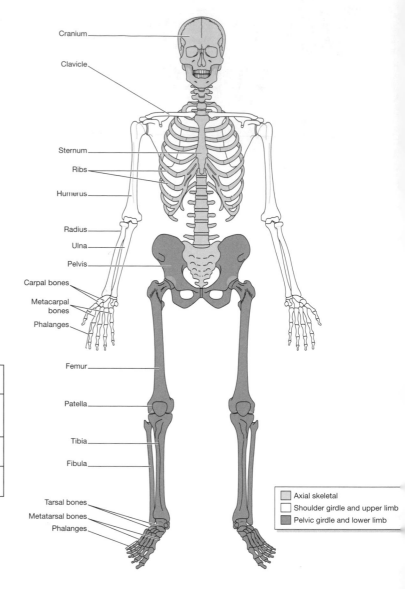

Figure 16.3

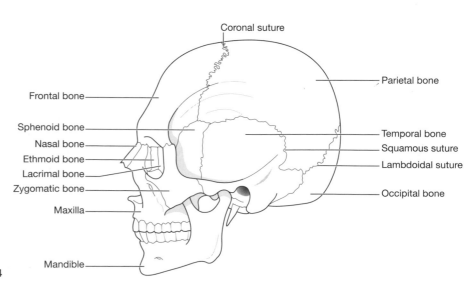

Figure 16.4

20. Sinuses contain **air** and are found in the **sphenoid, ethmoid, maxillary** and **frontal** bones. They all communicate with the **nasal cavity** and are lined with **ciliated epithelium**. Their functions are to give **resonance** to the voice and **lighten** the bones of the face and cranium.

Fontanelles are distinct **membranous** areas of the skull in infants and are present until **ossification** is complete and the skull bones fuse. The largest are the **anterior** fontanelle, present until **12–18** months, and the **posterior** fontanelle that usually closes over by **2–3** months of age. Their presence allows for moulding of the baby's **head** during childbirth.

21.

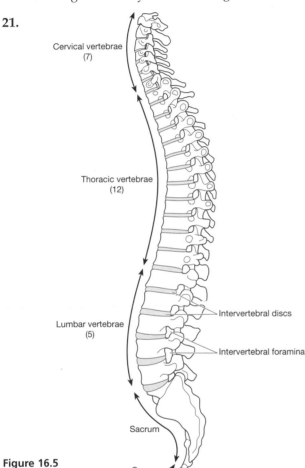

Figure 16.5

22. a. 7, b. 12, c. 5, d. 5, e. 4.

23.

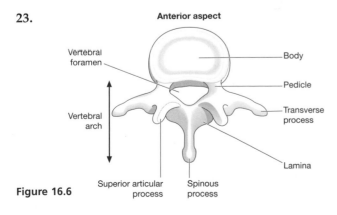

Figure 16.6

24. a. Coccyx; b. transverse foramen; c. thoracic vertebrae; d. atlas; e. axis; f. sacrum; g. odontoid process; h. vertebral foramen; i. intervertebral disc; j. annulus fibrosus; k. nucleus pulposus.

25.

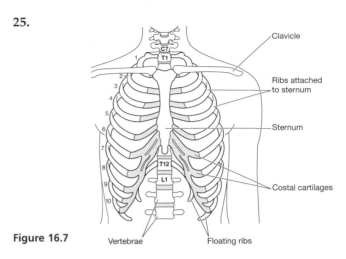

Figure 16.7

26. Intercostal nerves

27.

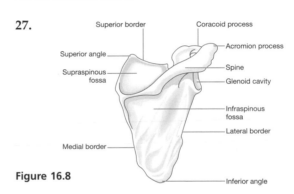

Figure 16.8

28.

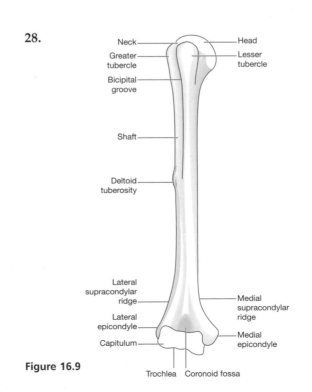

Figure 16.9

29. and 30.

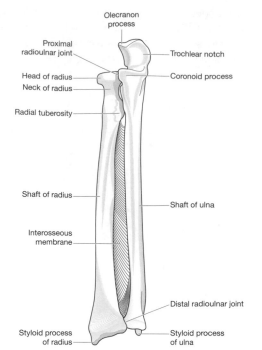

Figure 16.10

Olecranon process
Proximal radioulnar joint
Trochlear notch
Head of radius
Coronoid process
Neck of radius
Radial tuberosity
Shaft of radius
Shaft of ulna
Interosseous membrane
Distal radioulnar joint
Styloid process of radius
Styloid process of ulna

31. and 32.

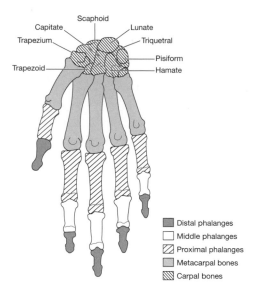

Figure 16.11

Scaphoid
Capitate
Lunate
Trapezium
Triquetral
Pisiform
Trapezoid
Hamate

Distal phalanges
Middle phalanges
Proximal phalanges
Metacarpal bones
Carpal bones

33. a. Humerus; b. scapula; c. ulna; d. scapula.

34. and 35.

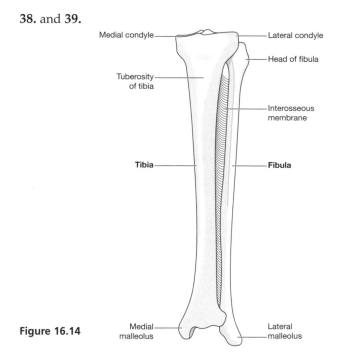

Figure 16.12

Iliac crest
Posterior
Anterior
Sciatic notch
Spine of ischium
Acetabulum with lines indicating joints
Ischial tuberosity
Symphysis pubis
Obturator foramen
Joint between ischium and pubis

Ilium
Ischium
Pubis

36. and 37.

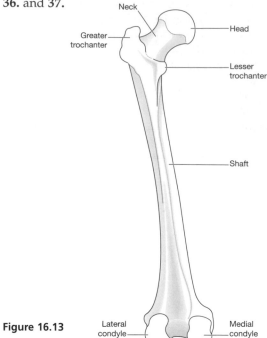

Figure 16.13

Neck
Head
Greater trochanter
Lesser trochanter
Shaft
Lateral condyle
Medial condyle

38. and 39.

Medial condyle
Lateral condyle
Head of fibula
Tuberosity of tibia
Interosseous membrane
Tibia
Fibula
Medial malleolus
Lateral malleolus

Figure 16.14

40. To stabilise and maintain the alignment of the tibia and fibula.

41. and 42.

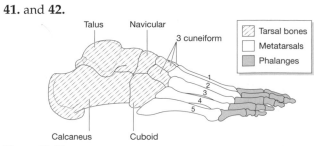

Talus
Navicular
3 cuneiform
Tarsal bones
Metatarsals
Phalanges
Calcaneus
Cuboid

Figure 16.15

43.

	Type (S, F or C)	Movement (I, Sl, Fr)
Suture	F	I
Tooth in jaw	C	I
Shoulder joint	S	Fr
Symphysis pubis	C	Sl
Knee joint	S	Fr
Interosseous membrane	F	Sl
Hip joint	S	Fr
Joint between phalanges	S	Fr
Intervertebral discs	C	Sl

Table 16.3. Joints and movements.

44. a. Flexion; b. extension; c. abduction; d. adduction; e. circumduction; f. rotation; g. pronation; h. supination; i. inversion; j. eversion.

45.

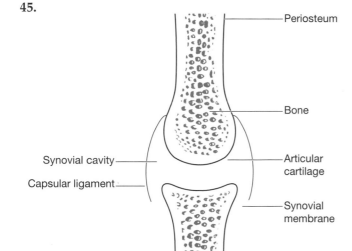

Figure 16.16

46. Provides nutrients for the structures within the joint cavity, protection as phagocytes remove microbes and cellular debris, lubricates, maintains joint stability, keeps the ends of the bones together.

47. a. Blend with capsule and provide extra stability.
b. Provide stability and allow movement when the muscle contracts.

48. and **49.**

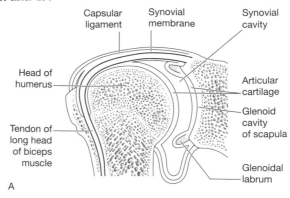

A

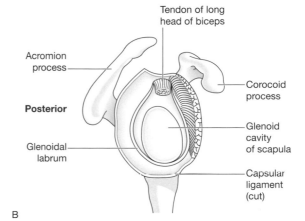

B

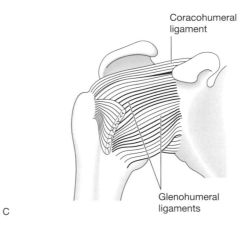

C

Figure 16.17

50. Ball and socket.

51. Table 16.4 Muscles involved in movement at the shoulder joint

Movement	Muscle(s) involved
Flexion	Coracobrachialis, anterior fibres of deltoid and pectoralis major
Extension	Teres major, latissimus dorsi, posterior deltoid
Abduction	Deltoid
Adduction	Combined action of flexors and extensors
Circumduction	Flexors, extensors, abductors and adductors
Medial rotation	Pectoralis major, latissimus dorsi, teres major, anterior deltoid
Lateral rotation	Posterior fibres of deltoid

52. Hinge

53. Table 16.5 Muscles involved in movement of the elbow

Movement	Muscle(s) involved
Flexion	Biceps, brachialis
Extension	Triceps

54. Hinge

55. Table 16.6 Muscles involved in movement of the proximal and distal radioulnar joints and wrist

Movement of radioulnar joints	Muscle(s) involved
Pronation	Pronator teres
Supination	Supinator, biceps
Movement of the wrist	
Flexion	Flexor carpi radialis, flexor carpi ulnaris
Extension	Extensor carpi radialis (longis and brevis), extensor carpi ulnaris
Abduction	Flexor and extensor carpi radialis
Adduction	Flexor and extensor carpi ulnaris

56. Ball and socket

57. and 58.

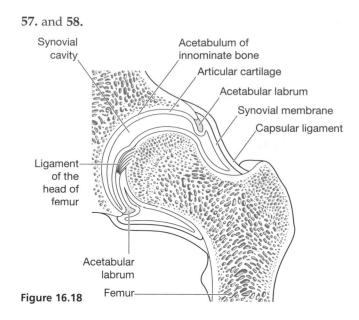

Figure 16.18

59. Table 16.7 Muscles involved in movement of the hip

Movement	Muscle(s) involved
Flexion	Psoas, iliacus, rectus femoris, sartorius
Extension	Gluteus maximus, hamstrings
Abduction	Gluteus medius and minimus, sartorius
Adduction	Adductor group
Medial rotation	Adductor group, gluteus medius and minimus
Lateral rotation	Quadriceps femoris, gluteus maximus, sartorius and, sometimes, adductor group

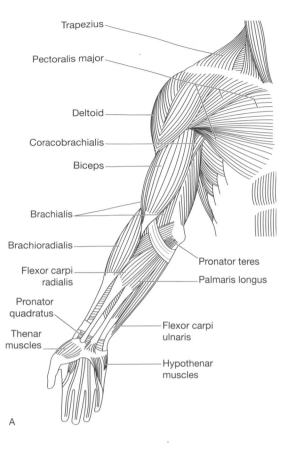

Trapezius
Pectoralis major
Deltoid
Coracobrachialis
Biceps
Brachialis
Brachioradialis
Flexor carpi radialis
Pronator teres
Palmaris longus
Pronator quadratus
Thenar muscles
Flexor carpi ulnaris
Hypothenar muscles

Trapezius
Deltoid
Teres minor
Teres major
Triceps
Latissimus dorsi
Brachioradialis
Extensor carpi radialis (longus and brevis)
Flexor carpi ulnaris
Extensor carpi ulnaris
Extensor digitorum

A   B

Figure 16.25

80.

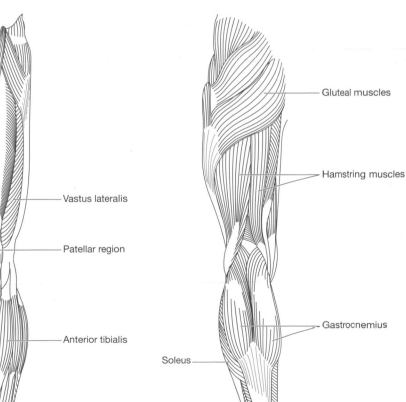

Iliacus
Psoas
Sartorius
Adductors of hip joint
Rectus femoris
Vastus lateralis
Vastus medialis
Patellar region
Patellar ligament (quadriceps tendon)
Gastrocnemius
Anterior tibialis
Soleus

Gluteal muscles
Hamstring muscles
Gastrocnemius
Soleus
Calcanean tendon

Figure 16.26   A   B

60 and **61.**

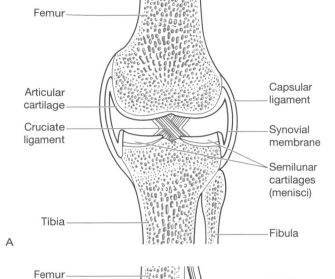

Femur
Articular cartilage
Cruciate ligament
Tibia
Capsular ligament
Synovial membrane
Semilunar cartilages (menisci)
Fibula

A

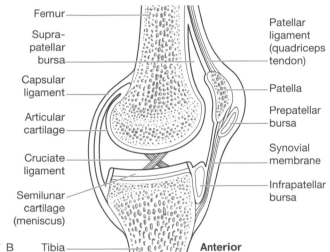

Femur
Supra-patellar bursa
Capsular ligament
Articular cartilage
Cruciate ligament
Semilunar cartilage (meniscus)
Patellar ligament (quadriceps tendon)
Patella
Prepatellar bursa
Synovial membrane
Infrapatellar bursa

B   Tibia   **Anterior**

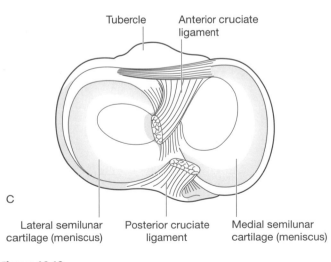

Tubercle   Anterior cruciate ligament

C

Lateral semilunar cartilage (meniscus)   Posterior cruciate ligament   Medial semilunar cartilage (meniscus)

Figure 16.19

62. Hinge

63. Table 16.8 Muscles involved in movement of the knee

Movement	Muscle(s) involved
Flexion	Gastrocnemius, hamstrings
Extension	Quadriceps femoris

64. Skeletal, cardiac and smooth muscle.

65.

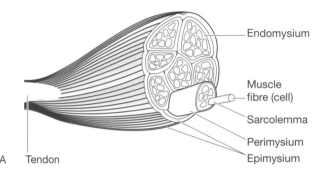

Endomysium
Muscle fibre (cell)
Sarcolemma
Perimysium
Epimysium

A   Tendon

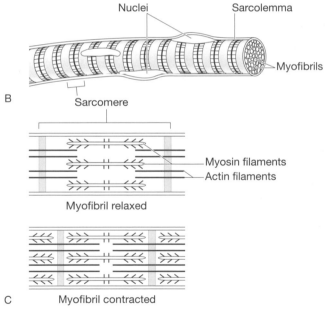

Nuclei   Sarcolemma
Myofibrils

B   Sarcomere

Myosin filaments
Actin filaments

Myofibril relaxed

C   Myofibril contracted

Figure 16.20

66. The functional unit of a skeletal muscle cell is the **sarcomere**. At each end of this unit are lines called **Z-lines**. Within the unit are two types of filament, thick filaments (made of **myosin**), and thin ones, made of **actin**. When the muscle cell is relaxed, these two filaments are not connected to each other. Contraction is initiated when an electrical impulse, called an **action potential**, passes along the cell membrane (also called the **sarcolemma**) of the muscle cell and penetrates deep into the sarcoplasm via the network of **channels** that run through the cell. This electrical stimulation causes **calcium** ions to be released from the **calcium stores** within the cell; these ions cause links, called **cross bridges** to form between the thick and thin filaments. The filaments pull on each other, which causes the functional unit to **shorten** in length, pulling the **Z-lines** at either end towards one another. If enough units are stimulated to contract at the same time, the entire **muscle** will also **shorten (contract)**.

67. The axons of motor neurones conveying impulses to skeletal muscles divide into fine filaments that end in motor end-plates. Each muscle fibre is stimulated at one motor end-plate and one motor nerve has many motor end-plates. The nerve impulse is passed across the neuromuscular junction – the gap between the motor end-plate and the muscle fibre – by the neurotransmitter acetylcholine. The group of muscle fibres and the motor end-plates of the nerve fibres that supply them form a motor unit.

68.

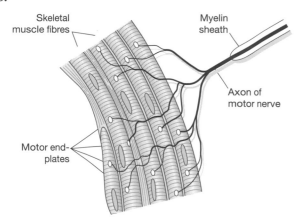

Figure 16.21

69. Muscle work with shortening of muscle
70. Muscle work with no shortening of muscle but increased tension developed, as when trying to lift an immovable load
71. The (usually proximal) attachment point of a muscle, which usually remains steady when the muscle contracts
72. Increase in size of muscle, due to enlargement of individual muscle fibres
73. Two muscles that work in opposition to each other across one or more joints.

74.

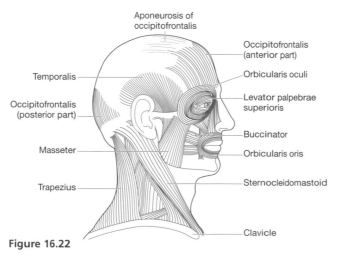

Figure 16.22

75. Table 16.9 Functions of muscles of the face and neck

Muscle	Paired/unpaired	Function
Occipitofrontalis	Unpaired	Raises the eyebrows
Levator palpebrae superioris	Paired	Raise the eyelids
Orbicularis oculi	Paired	Close the eyes and screws them up
Buccinator	Paired	Draw in the cheeks and expels air forcibly
Orbicularis oris	Unpaired	Closes the lips and involved in whistling
Masseter	Paired	Draw the mandible up to the maxilla for chewing
Temporalis	Paired	Close the mouth and involved in chewing
Pterygoid	Paired	Close the mouth and pulls the lower jaw forwards
Sternocleidomastoid	Paired	Contraction of one: draws the head towards the shoulder Contraction of both: flexion of the cervical vertebrae draw sternum and clavicles upwards
Trapezius	Paired	Pull the head backwards, squares the shoulders and controls movements of the scapula when the shoulder is in use

76.

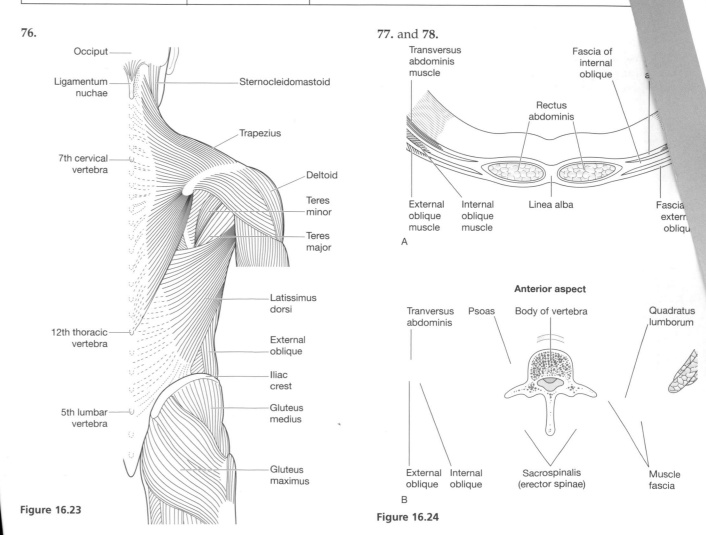

Figure 16.23

77. and 78.

Figure 16.24

60 and **61.**

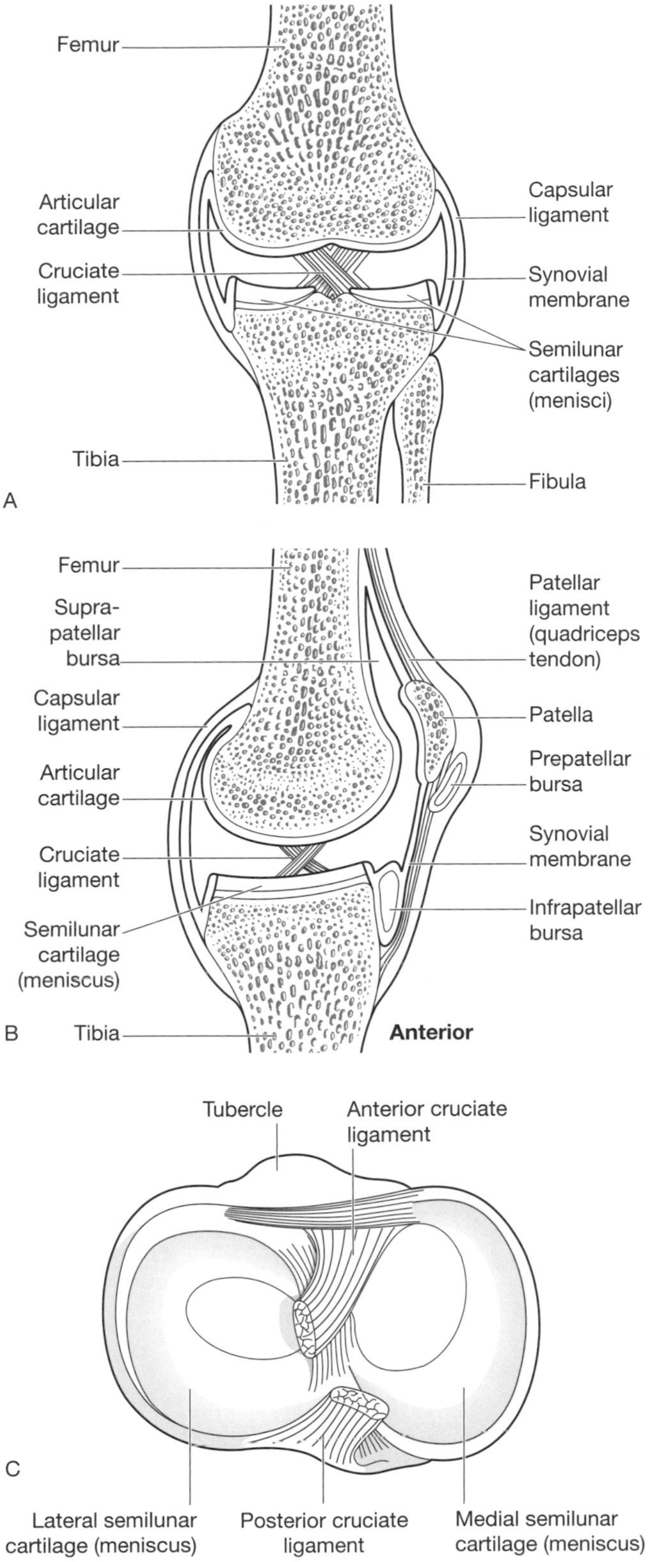

Femur

Articular
cartilage

Cruciate
ligament

Tibia

A

Capsular
ligament

Synovial
membrane

Semilunar
cartilages
(menisci)

Fibula

Femur

Supra-
patellar
bursa

Capsular
ligament

Articular
cartilage

Cruciate
ligament

Semilunar
cartilage
(meniscus)

B   Tibia

Patellar
ligament
(quadriceps
tendon)

Patella

Prepatellar
bursa

Synovial
membrane

Infrapatellar
bursa

Anterior

Tubercle   Anterior cruciate
ligament

C

Lateral semilunar
cartilage (meniscus)

Posterior cruciate
ligament

Medial semilunar
cartilage (meniscus)

Figure 16.19

62. Hinge

63. Table 16.8 Muscles involved in movement of the knee

Movement	Muscle(s) involved
Flexion	Gastrocnemius, hamstrings
Extension	Quadriceps femoris

64. Skeletal, cardiac and smooth muscle.

65.

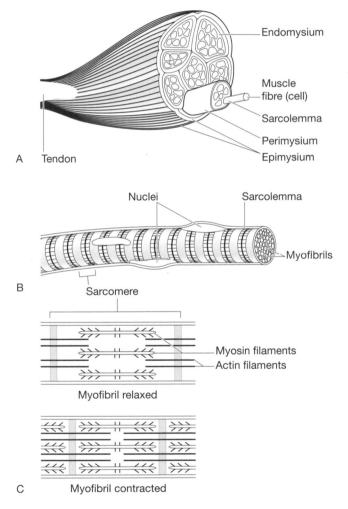

A   Tendon

Endomysium

Muscle
fibre (cell)

Sarcolemma

Perimysium
Epimysium

Nuclei   Sarcolemma

B

Myofibrils

Sarcomere

Myosin filaments
Actin filaments

Myofibril relaxed

C   Myofibril contracted

Figure 16.20

66. The functional unit of a skeletal muscle cell is the **sarcomere**. At each end of this unit are lines called **Z-lines**. Within the unit are two types of filament, thick filaments (made of **myosin**), and thin ones, made of **actin**. When the muscle cell is relaxed, these two filaments are not connected to each other. Contraction is initiated when an electrical impulse, called an **action potential**, passes along the cell membrane (also called the **sarcolemma**) of the muscle cell and penetrates deep into the sarcoplasm via the network of **channels** that run through the cell. This electrical stimulation causes **calcium** ions to be released from the **calcium stores** within the cell; these ions cause links, called **cross bridges** to form between the thick and thin filaments. The filaments pull on each other, which causes the functional unit to **shorten** in length, pulling the **Z-lines** at either end towards one another. If enough units are stimulated to contract at the same time, the entire **muscle** will also **shorten (contract)**.

67. The axons of motor neurones conveying impulses to skeletal muscles divide into fine filaments that end in motor end-plates. Each muscle fibre is stimulated at one motor end-plate and one motor nerve has many motor end-plates. The nerve impulse is passed across the neuromuscular junction – the gap between the motor end-plate and the muscle fibre – by the neurotransmitter acetylcholine. The group of muscle fibres and the motor end-plates of the nerve fibres that supply them form a motor unit.

68.

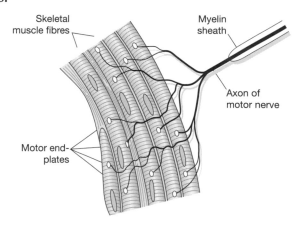

Figure 16.21

69. Muscle work with shortening of muscle

70. Muscle work with no shortening of muscle but increased tension developed, as when trying to lift an immovable load

71. The (usually proximal) attachment point of a muscle, which usually remains steady when the muscle contracts

72. Increase in size of muscle, due to enlargement of individual muscle fibres

73. Two muscles that work in opposition to each other across one or more joints.

74.

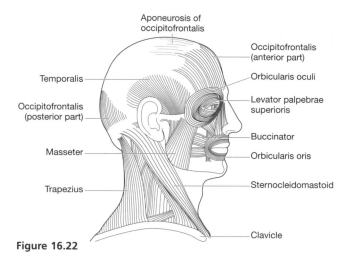

Figure 16.22

75. Table 16.9 Functions of muscles of the face and neck

Muscle	Paired/unpaired	Function
Occipitofrontalis	Unpaired	Raises the eyebrows
Levator palpebrae superioris	Paired	Raise the eyelids
Orbicularis oculi	Paired	Close the eyes and screws them up
Buccinator	Paired	Draw in the cheeks and expels air forcibly
Orbicularis oris	Unpaired	Closes the lips and involved in whistling
Masseter	Paired	Draw the mandible up to the maxilla for chewing
Temporalis	Paired	Close the mouth and involved in chewing
Pterygoid	Paired	Close the mouth and pulls the lower jaw forwards
Sternocleidomastoid	Paired	Contraction of one: draws the head towards the shoulder Contraction of both: flexion of the cervical vertebrae drawing the sternum and clavicles upwards
Trapezius	Paired	Pull the head backwards, squares the shoulders and controls movements of the scapula when the shoulder is in use

76.

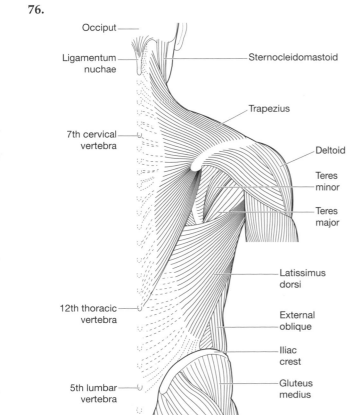

Occiput
Ligamentum nuchae
Sternocleidomastoid
Trapezius
7th cervical vertebra
Deltoid
Teres minor
Teres major
12th thoracic vertebra
Latissimus dorsi
External oblique
Iliac crest
5th lumbar vertebra
Gluteus medius
Gluteus maximus

Figure 16.23

77. and 78.

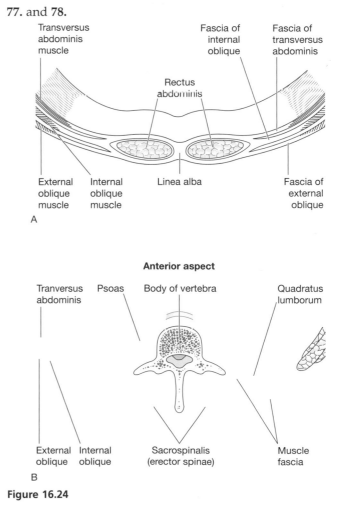

Transversus abdominis muscle
Fascia of internal oblique
Fascia of transversus abdominis
Rectus abdominis
External oblique muscle
Internal oblique muscle
Linea alba
Fascia of external oblique

A

Anterior aspect

Tranversus abdominis
Psoas
Body of vertebra
Quadratus lumborum
External oblique
Internal oblique
Sacrospinalis (erector spinae)
Muscle fascia

B

Figure 16.24

79.

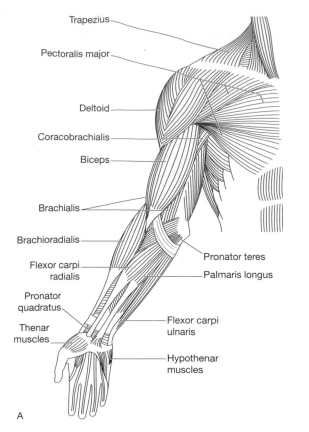

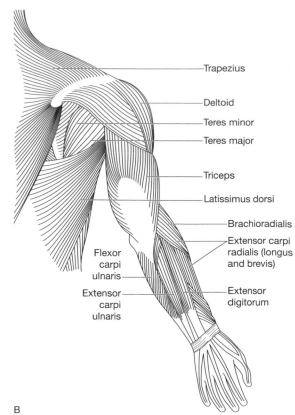

Figure 16.25   A   B

80.

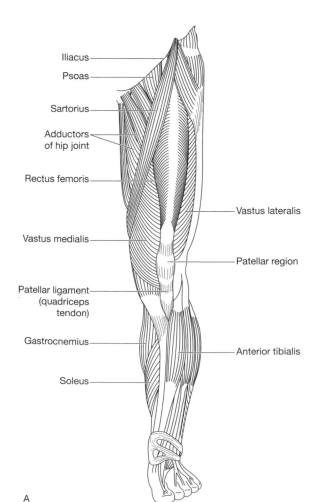

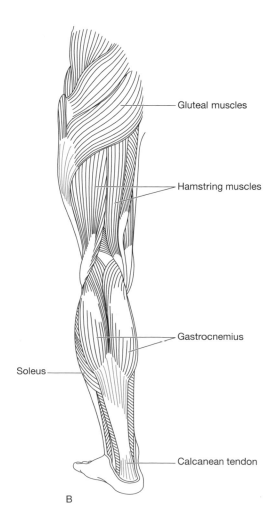

Figure 16.26   A   B

81.

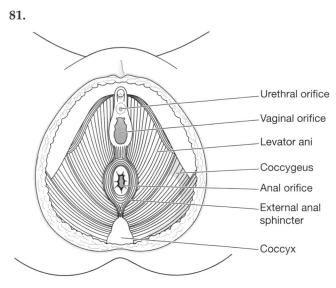

Urethral orifice

Vaginal orifice

Levator ani

Coccygeus

Anal orifice

External anal sphincter

Coccyx

Figure 16.27

82. It acts as a support for the organs of the pelvis and maintains continence by resisting raised intrapelvic pressure during micturition and defaecation.

17 Introduction to genetics

ANSWERS

1. c   2. c   3. d   4. a   7 and 8.

5. a. Deoxyribonucleic acid.   b. Ribonucleic acid.

6. The nucleus contains the body's **genetic** material, in the form of DNA, which is built from nucleotides, each made up of three components: a **phosphate** group, the sugar **deoxyribose** and one of four **bases**. DNA is a double strand of nucleotides that resembles a **helix**, or twisted ladder. DNA and associated proteins, also called **histones**, are coiled together, forming **chromatin**. During cell division, the DNA becomes very tightly coiled and can be seen as **chromosomes** under the microscope. There are **23** pairs of them in most human cells. Each consists of many functional subunits called **genes**. Any given type of cell uses only part of the whole genetic code, also called the **genome**, to carry out its specific activities. Each **gene** contains the genetic code, or instructions, for the synthesis of one **protein**, that could, for example, be an **enzyme** needed to catalyse a particular chemical **reaction**, a hormone, or it may form part of the structure of a cell. The coded instructions have to be transferred to the **cytoplasm** of the cell, since that is where the organelles that make protein, the **ribosomes**, are found. DNA itself does not transfer, but a copy of the genetic code is made in the form of **mRNA**, which leaves the **nucleus**. When its instructions have been read and the new protein synthesised, the copy is destroyed.

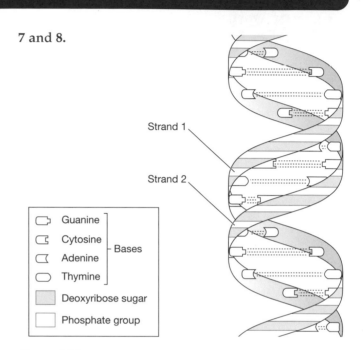

Figure 17.1

9.

Table 17.1

DNA Strand 1	C	C	G	T	A	A	C	T	C	A	A	T	G	T
DNA Strand 2	G	G	C	A	T	T	G	A	G	T	T	A	C	A
mRNA	G	G	C	A	U	U	G	A	G	U	U	A	C	A

10.

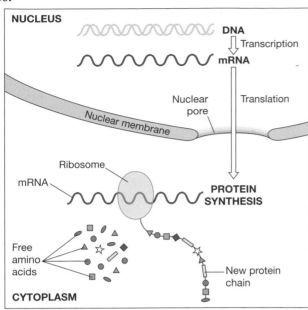

Figure 17.2

11. **a.** RNA   **b.** DNA   **c.** both   **d.** RNA
    e. DNA   **f.** RNA   **g.** RNA   **h.** RNA
    i. both   **j.** DNA

12. **a.** Translation takes place on the ribosomes in the cytoplasm.

    b. True

    c. A codon is a piece of RNA carrying information

    d. True

    e. Some new proteins are made for export, e.g. insulin

    f. Red blood cells have no nucleus, and gametes carry only half

    g. True

    h. True

13.

Table 17.2

	Mitosis	Meiosis
One division or two?	One	Two
Daughter cells diploid or haploid?	Diploid	Haploid
Does crossing over take place?	No	Yes
Are daughter cells identical to parent?	Yes	No
Two or four cells produced?	Two	Four
Are daughter cells identical to one another?	Yes	No
Which process produces gametes?	–	Yes
Which process replaces damaged cells?	Yes	–

14. One chromosome of each pair is inherited from the mother and one from the father, so there are **two** copies of each gene in the cell. Two chromosomes of the same pair are called **homologues**, and the genes are present in paired sites called **alleles**.

    When the paired genes are identical, they are called **homozygous**, but if they are different forms they are called **heterozygous**. Dominant genes are always **expressed over recessive genes**. Individuals homozygous for a dominant gene **cannot** pass the recessive form on to their children, and individuals heterozygous for a gene **can** pass on either form of the gene to theirs.

15. Expression of genes in an individual, e.g. blue eyed or brown haired.

16. The genes present on an individual's chromosomes. Dominant genes are usually represented by a capital letter, recessive with the corresponding lower case letter.

17.

Box 17.1

	T	t
T	TT	Tt
t	Tt	tt

18. TT and Tt

19. TT and tt

20.

Box 17.2

	B	B
b	Bb	Bb
b	Bb	Bb

21. None (no bb)

22.

Box 17.3

	X^B	Y
X^b	$X^B X^b$	$X^b Y$
X^b	$X^B X^b$	$X^b Y$

23. 50:50

24. 100% (both of them)

25. Carriers

18 | The reproductive system

ANSWERS

1. and 2.

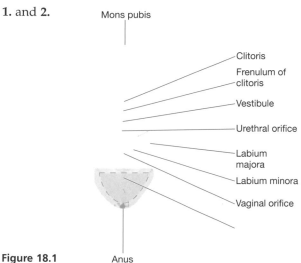

Mons pubis

Clitoris
Frenulum of clitoris
Vestibule
Urethral orifice
Labium majora
Labium minora
Vaginal orifice

Figure 18.1   Anus

3. and 4.

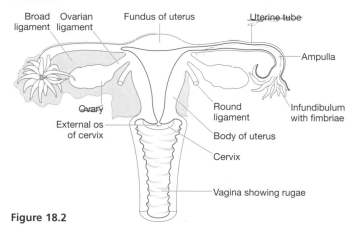

Broad ligament
Ovarian ligament
Fundus of uterus
Uterine tube
Ampulla
Ovary
External os of cervix
Round ligament
Infundibulum with fimbriae
Body of uterus
Cervix
Vagina showing rugae

Figure 18.2

5. and 6.

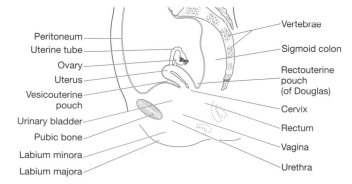

Peritoneum
Uterine tube
Ovary
Uterus
Vesicouterine pouch
Urinary bladder
Pubic bone
Labium minora
Labium majora

Vertebrae
Sigmoid colon
Rectouterine pouch (of Douglas)
Cervix
Rectum
Vagina
Urethra

Figure 18.3

7.
In the vagina, where the acid environment protects against ascending infection.

8. and 9.

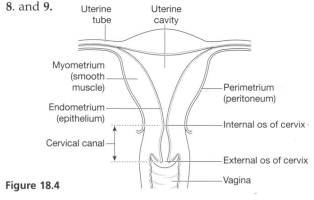

Uterine tube
Uterine cavity
Myometrium (smooth muscle)
Endometrium (epithelium)
Cervical canal
Perimetrium (peritoneum)
Internal os of cervix
External os of cervix
Vagina

Figure 18.4

10. b.   **11.** a., b., c.   **12.** c., d.   **13.** a., c., d.

14., 15., 16., 17.

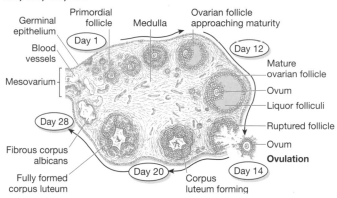

Germinal epithelium
Blood vessels
Mesovarium
Day 1
Day 28
Fibrous corpus albicans
Fully formed corpus luteum
Day 20
Primordial follicle
Medulla
Day 12
Ovarian follicle approaching maturity
Mature ovarian follicle
Ovum
Liquor folliculi
Ruptured follicle
Ovum
Ovulation
Day 14
Corpus luteum forming

Figure 18.5

18. Maturation of the follicle is stimulated by **follicle stimulating hormone** released by the anterior pituitary, and oestrogen from the **follicular cells**. Ovulation is triggered by a surge of **luteinizing hormone**, which is secreted by the anterior pituitary. This release takes place a few **hours** before ovulation. After ovulation, the now empty follicle develops into the **corpus luteum**, and its main function is to secrete **progesterone and oestrogen**, which maintains the uterine lining in case fertilization and implantation occur. If pregnancy does occur, the embedded ovum supports the corpus luteum by producing **human chorionic gonadotrophin**, which keeps it functioning for the next 3 months or so, until the **placenta** is developed enough to take on this role. If pregnancy does not occur, the corpus luteum degenerates and forms a scar on the surface of the ovary called the **corpus albicans**.

19. Maturation of the uterus, uterine tubes and ovaries; beginning of the menstrual cycle; development of the breasts; growth of pubic and axillary hair; increase in body height and pelvic width; deposition of subcutaneous fat, especially at hips and breasts.

20.

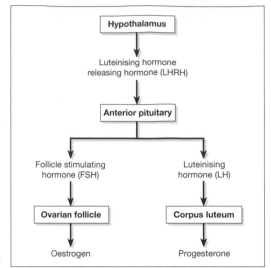

Figure 18.6

21. a. LHRH from the hypothalamus causes anterior pituitary secretion of FSH and LH.
b. FSH promotes ovarian follicular development and follicular secretion of oestrogen in the first half of the menstrual cycle.
c. LH triggers ovulation, and stimulates development of the corpus luteum, which synthesizes progesterone.
d. Oestrogen stimulates the development of the female secondary sexual characteristics at puberty, stimulates breast growth in pregnancy, stimulates proliferation of the endometrium in the first half of the menstrual cycle, and with progesterone, turns off LH and FSH production in the second half of the menstrual cycle (so that another ovum is not released until after menstruation).
e. Progesterone with oestrogen promotes sexual changes at puberty; with oestrogen it regulates FSH and LH levels in the second half of the menstrual cycle; it maintains the thick vascular lining of the uterus in the second half of the menstrual cycle and during pregnancy and prevents menstruation.

22. and 23. (See Figure 18.7.)

24. Anterior pituitary.

25. Ovulation (event E) is caused by the sudden surge in the levels of LH.

26. See the answer version of Figure 18.7.

27. Progesterone.

28. See the answer version of Figure 18.7.

29. They are being synthesized by the corpus luteum, which will begin to degenerate in the absence of pregnancy, and therefore oestrogen and progesterone levels will start to decline.

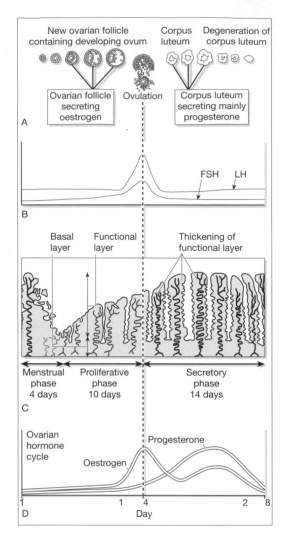

Figure 18.7

30. If pregnancy occurs, the developing embryo secretes human chorionic gonadotrophin (hCG), which maintains the corpus luteum for 3–4 months; during this time it continues to secrete oestrogen and progesterone (on which the pregnancy depends). At the end of this time, the placenta is mature enough to maintain oestrogen and progesterone levels.

31.

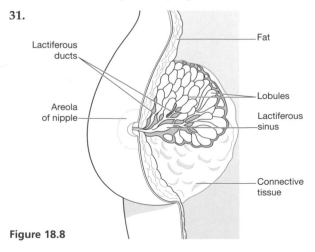

Figure 18.8

32. Table 18.1 The effect of hormones on the breast

Statement	Hormone(s)
Stimulates body growth and development in puberty	Oestrogen and progesterone
Initiates release of milk	Oxytocin
Stimulates production of milk	Prolactin
Stimulates growth and development in pregnancy	Oestrogen and progesterone

33. and 34.

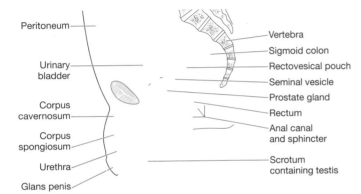

Figure 18.9

35., 36. and 37. (See Figure 18.10)

38. c.   **39.** d.   **40.** b.   **41.** d.   **42.** b.

43.

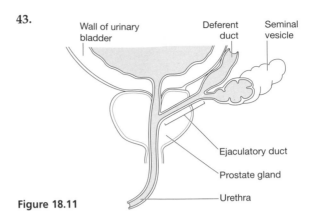

Figure 18.11

44. Table 18.2 Nature and function of sperm volume

	% sperm volume	Function
Spermatozoa	10	Sex cells to fertilize the ovum
Prostate secretions	30	Clotting enzyme to thicken sperm and increase the likelihood of sperm pooling at the cervix
Seminal vesicle secretions	60	Contain nutrients such as glucose to nourish sperm on their journey into the vagina; slightly alkaline to protect sperm from acid secretions of vagina

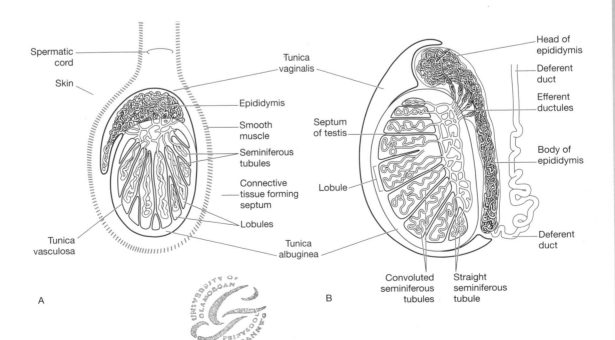

Figure 18.10